High Percentage
Wellness
Steps

Suneel Dhand, M.D.

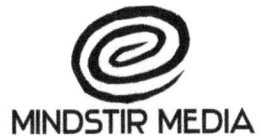

High Percentage Wellness Steps
Copyright © 2011 by Suneel Dhand, M.D. All rights reserved.

No part of this book may be used or reproduced in any manner whatsoever without written permission, except in the case of brief quotations embodied in critical articles and reviews. For more information, e-mail all inquiries to:
info@mindstirmedia.com

Published by Mindstir Media
PO Box 1681 | Hampton, New Hampshire 03843 | USA
1.800.767.0531 | www.mindstirmedia.com

Printed in the United States of America

ISBN-10: 0-981964-87-7
ISBN-13: 978-0-9819648-7-4

Library of Congress Control Number: 2011928133

Visit Suneel Dhand, M.D. on the World Wide Web:
www.suneeldhand.com

To my parents, without whom no achievement in my life would be possible, and to whom I owe everything that is best in me.

INTRODUCTION

"How are you today?" This is a standard greeting we all give to each other, be it with family, friends, colleagues or a complete stranger. By reflex, most of us will immediately say something along the lines of "I'm well, thanks," or "Doing good." It's rare for us to say, "I feel horrible," or "I'm not good," even if we are having a truly terrible day! We are by default always "well" and it seems as if we are programmed to answer this way. So, if this is the most common question asked of us, then what exactly is this thing called wellness that folks are inquiring about?

The World Health Organization defines wellness as "a state of complete physical, mental and social well-being and not merely the absence of disease or infirmity." Clearly then, while the absence of illness can be argued to be the most important factor, it is not all that matters when we talk about wellness. Can somebody suffering from many medical illnesses be perceived to be more well than someone who doesn't? The answer is, emphatically, *yes*. I have seen wheelchair-bound patients suffering from the most terrible illnesses, who—on the face of it, and certainly in the way they project themselves—appear more well than some of my patients who have relatively minor issues.

Here's a little exercise for you to perform. Close your eyes for ten seconds and think about the healthiest and most well people you know. What is it about them that makes you perceive them that way? Are they in great shape? Are they lucky enough to not suffer from any illnesses? Do they stick to a good diet? Do they know how to handle stress well? Are they positive people with a great outlook? The answer is likely a combination of these factors. Wellness and well-being, therefore, encompass a whole host of physical, emotional and social factors.

In my everyday practice as a physician, I encounter patients with a vast array of conditions, from asthma and high blood pressure, to heart attacks and strokes. As doctors we are trained to identify and treat disease processes which, of course, is the focus of our daily efforts. Medical students learn to recognize symptoms and signs and what tests to order. When doctors read the test results, they know instantly what other investigations to do, what medicine to prescribe, or which specialist to call upon. We are taught to take full advantage of the wonders of modern medicine to cure illness. In countless years spent in medical school and training, through all those lectures and late nights of study, surprisingly little time, however, was spent learning the basics of health and wellness, and the underlying concepts that determine these. We would learn all about a certain disease and how to treat it, but very little about the simple preventive practices that may reduce the chances of it arising in the first place. We are not taught to talk to patients about their whole lifestyle and daily practices that determine their complete well-being. Posters and pamphlets are sometimes given out, but how many physicians spend even a few minutes talking to their patients about wellness and prevention? Unfortunately, not that many. Seeing the lack of education in this area, and the tremendous potential for improvement, led to my interest in wellness and preventive medicine. The power of simply telling a patient to increase his or her fiber intake or exercise every day—not just as a passing piece of advice, but as a convincing argument based on solid science—is a unique position for a physician to be in. Unfortunately, most doctors feel under tremendous time pressure or believe that other health professionals such as nurses or dietitians can address these issues with the patient.

Another problem in the wellness debate is that we as doctors too often think that we are only in the business of alleviating suffering and returning our patients to the same "zero baseline" they had before they became ill. Why not go the other way and try to improve that initial baseline? This is the problem with modern medical philosophy in general. We never try hard enough to actively *increase* well-being.

Patients and families often ask me what else they can do, aside from taking their medicines, to help them with their general health. This is where doctors fall down, and rarely give detailed advice. In recent years there has been a large amount of research looking into preventive medicine and the power of simple lifestyle changes to bring about positive substantial changes in our lives. I am writing this book to show you some of this overwhelming evidence, and help you incorporate these practices into your daily routine. All of us have heard the familiar themes about eating more fruit, exercising more, de-stressing and staying positive—but what exactly do the scientific studies say? These mantras are not just bumper stickers. The funny thing is that a lot of this evidence-based research is common knowledge based on our own experiences. We all know intuitively that when we eat a high-fat meal we don't feel as well as we would after a healthy meal. We know that after exercise we get a natural boost. We all know that being in nature helps us de-stress. As we all learned in history class, *we hold these truths to be self-evident.* But what seems to be common sense to many of us isn't always followed. Simply knowing what to do, apparently, is not enough.

There can, of course, never be any guarantee of health and wellness. We've all heard the stories of Uncle Joe who "ate well and exercised his whole life and still got sick." Anyone can be unlucky, and the most well-reputed fitness enthusiasts and healthy athletes can all get sick too. But the point is that Uncle Joe led a much healthier life beforehand, and as a result would also have been in a better position to get through his sickness because he had a solid foundation beforehand.

Most of us have a great knack for understanding percentages, probably because we all went to school and anxiously received our grades this way! I always ask my patients when they are recovering from an illness, "How much, as a percentage, do you feel like yourself?" The patient will often say to me, "Doc, I feel 50 percent better," "I feel 80 percent better," or if it's a bad day, "Doc, I feel 20 percent worse!" I put it to you, next time you interact with your doctors, turn the question around and ask *them* when they give you a treatment what the percentage is that you will experience benefit. Do this *before* you sign the consent form or swallow that pill.

As I watch the latest commercial or read an article on a wonderful new medication or treatment that has just been released, I often like to dig a little deeper into the statistics. Many of these new drugs or procedures are tested thoroughly in research studies and, at best, show a 5 to 10 percent improvement over a placebo, which is an "empty" pill, often containing something like sugar. A surprising number of new treatments are hailed as successes when they show only a small percentage difference in outcome. In fact, statistically speaking, a study treatment can have a "number needed to treat" of over 20 and still be judged reasonably effective. That means that under one in 20 people (5 percent) will likely experience any benefit. Think about that. If you were presented with that statistic, you probably wouldn't fancy your chances too much. Some of these treatments cost thousands of dollars a year too. What if you could choose between one of these medications, or a simple lifestyle change that could improve your health by a potentially much higher percentage? Of course, the lifestyle change is harder (although much cheaper), but which one sounds more promising and more beneficial? This is not meant to discount the miracles of modern medicine, without which we would all be past our life expectancy by our thirties, and would constantly be on the lookout for the next deadly plague. New drugs and treatments have transformed mankind in unbelievable ways over the last 100 years, and I am proud to practice evidence-based modern medicine. That being said, a massive amount of illness now is largely a result of the choices we make and the lifestyles we lead. In other words, easily *preventable* illnesses.

I have written this book to show you some easy, natural steps which can make huge differences to your health and wellness. I have tried to make everything as simple and straightforward as possible, avoiding a lot of detailed medical jargon. I've seen many books that go into excessive scientific detail and analysis, but I wanted to make this as basic and readable as possible. Many of the studies you are about to read about have much higher percentage improvements than those with new expensive treatments—percentages the medical community would be raving about if it were a new drug or invasive procedure that had just been approved. You may notice in some of the latter chapters that many of the studies do not present their results in classic percentage terms, purely because the types of experiments being performed are measuring subjective qualities like stress and happiness, which obviously can't be measured directly in percentage terms. Nevertheless, the basic premise is the same in looking at proven measures to improve our well-being.

So you will be taken through some key high percentage steps to your wellness. Seven key pillars that relate to areas that are among the most problematic in society and cause the most ill-being, both physical and emotional. As you read, you will see how they are all interlinked with each other, to form the basis of your complete well-being. All the things which, when combined, truly give you the best chance of meaning it the next time you answer the question, "How are you?," by saying, "I feel well!"

RECOMMENDATIONS IN THIS BOOK ARE BASED ON AVAILABLE SCIENTIFIC EVIDENCE. THIS IS NOT A SUBSTITUTE FOR ANY MEDICAL ADVICE GIVEN BY YOUR OWN PHYSICIAN, WHOM YOU SHOULD ALWAYS CONSULT BEFORE INTRODUCING ANY MAJOR CHANGES TO YOUR LIFESTYLE.

CHAPTER ONE

NUTRITION WELLNESS: EVIDENCE-BASED EATING

Food is the fuel that nourishes and sustains us. Everything our body does, whether it's growing, replenishing, moving or thinking, requires energy. What we eat, therefore, not only determines our weight and body shape, but also our energy levels, mood, logic and intelligence. It is the first cornerstone of our health and wellness. To use the time-honored cliché, we are what we eat. If we aren't consuming the right nutrients, there is no way that we can function at our full potential and achieve maximum well-being. We've all been in a position where we haven't eaten for a while and find ourselves consumed with hunger. During these troughs we are not at any imminent risk of starvation, but we are not able to think straight and often find ourselves irritable and somewhat irrational. As the old saying goes, *a hungry man is an angry man*, and it's very true. Fortunately, any hunger we experience in America is, for most of us, a brief, transient issue that is quickly resolved when we have the opportunity to eat. We are lucky to live in a country where the main problem is abundance rather than scarcity. Our problem is, in fact, that we as a nation substantially overeat, in addition to being addicted to the wrong types of foods.

For too many of us, sticking to a healthier diet is a temporary measure when we feel guilty about how much we've been eating or are trying desperately to get into shape for that special occasion—whether it's a birthday party, wedding, graduation, or class reunion. After that special occasion, though, we often quickly go back to our old habits. That is the wrong way to go about things. Eating well is a lifestyle habit that involves a consistent nutrition pattern. It's your own unique relationship to what you eat every day. There's also a misconception that healthy eating involves terrible sacrifices, and means eating boring, dull and tasteless food. Nothing could be further from the truth. There are a wealth of delicious, satisfying and healthy foods to choose from.

None of us would ever dream of deliberately pouring detergent or paint into our car's fuel tank, or going to an unreliable mechanic. We take so much care to look for a decent gas station. If it looks dingy or doesn't have a reliable company behind it, we will think twice about filling up our car at that location! If we take so much care of our car, why then do we put food into our own bodies that is potentially detrimental and does us no good? All it takes is a little pause to think before we eat, in order to make better choices.

Our addiction to high-calorie foods

Before we even get into the debate about what to eat, the simple fact is that, in general, we simply eat too much! It is inherent in our culture. Every other restaurant offers a great value buffet, where we are encouraged to eat as much as possible and load up our plate at least three or four times. Then we're seduced with the dessert menu. Even at home, it's all too easy to grab that bag of candies or chips to munch on while we are watching television. The temptations are always at hand. Don't get me wrong, I enjoy a good buffet as much as the next person, and I love dessert, too. Splurging once in a while is great fun—as long as it is a special treat. Many experts will tell you to avoid treats at all costs, but I disagree. Some even tell you to continue a strict diet over Thanksgiving or Christmas. But following a healthy eating plan doesn't have to be that harsh. Life would be dull if we didn't have some indulgences every now and again. Where we go wrong, however, is that too many times we treat ourselves too much. The transition from special treat to habit can be a subtle one.

The concept of a calorie is actually derived from physics, and is scientifically defined as the energy required to raise the temperature of one gram of water by one degree Celsius. Nowadays, this term is almost exclusively used to measure the amount of energy we are taking in via food. Each of us has our own basic requirement that varies according to our age, gender, body size and baseline activity levels. As a rough guide, an average young, active adult male will require about 2,500 calories a day, and a female, 2,000 calories a day. For many of us though, our caloric needs are even less. There are many online calculators available that can help you work out how many calories you really need. Use a search engine to find one and then plug in your own numbers.

As a reflection of our changing relationship with food, in the 1970s the average American male consumed 2,200 calories a day. By the 2000s, according to government statistics, that figure stood at a whopping 2,700 calories a day.[1] That's almost a 25 percent increase. Factor in that we are now less physically active than we used to be (modern inventions like computers do have their drawbacks), and you can see how this becomes a problem.

Take a look at the following foods, with their estimated potential calorie counts:

• Large slice of cheesecake: 500 calories

• Large coffee with whipped cream: 600 calories

• Double cheeseburger: 1,500 calories

• Large cheese fries: 2,000 calories

These calorie counts obviously depend on the size, portion and where you purchase your food, but for one food item to contain your entire daily allowance of calories is truly shocking. Yet, we love a lot of these foods!

Blame your inner caveman

One theory of our attraction to high-calorie foods goes back to our caveman days. Genetically, we are identical to those first humans who spent most of their lives scouring the land in pursuit of food for themselves and their families. Our caveman ancestor did not have the chance to step out to a nice restaurant for dinner or go to the fast food restaurant on the way home from work. Back then, we were dependent on high-calorie foods for survival, since they were a great source of energy to keep us going when we didn't know where or when our next meal would be. Hence, those foods were the right (and pretty much only) choice at that time. The problem is that we've now moved on from that jungle life and don't need to be so enamored with such foods any longer. But because our genetic make-up remains the same, something in us still keeps telling us to go ahead and gorge when we have the opportunity, especially when we are hungry.

Cutting down on calories if you overeat is the first step towards better health. On a recent trip I took to Europe, our tour group was walking in Paris when we were contemplating getting something to eat. One American member of the group turned to me and recalled that he hadn't eaten much lunch that day, saying, "The less I eat, the better I feel." He must have been comparing this to our other usual tour days when we would stop at a nice restaurant to eat a substantial lunch. I thought that what he said was very interesting. When we overeat, it can make us feel sluggish, lethargic and generally not as well as we would had we eaten less. More about that in a future chapter.

Scientific studies show that controlling caloric intake can have significant benefits. A large body of evidence even suggests that calorie restriction has an anti-aging effect, extending life span and reducing chronic disease in a number of different animals. In one interesting study, researchers studied the impact of dietary restriction on aging in mice.[2] The mice were divided into six groups that consumed different diets, from as much food as they wanted, to up to 65 percent calorie restriction. The results were startling. The mice from the restricted groups lived an impressive *35 to 65 percent longer* than the mice on higher calorie diets. The most calorie-restricted mice lived the longest of all, and the scientists were shocked to see that some of them even lived longer than any known mice they had studied before. These mice had better body weight and were also found to have improved immunity. A similar trend has been shown in other studies, with scientists concluding that calorie restriction has beneficial effects on metabolism, as well as slowing down cell damage, both of which result in a slower rate of aging. Does this mean that humans should severely restrict themselves too? Probably not, as this degree of caloric limitation is not only hard to maintain but can be dangerous as well. But such findings should give us food for thought (no pun intended) when most of us routinely consume more calories than we need on an everyday basis.

It is easy for us today to find out the calorie counts of most foods we eat. We can either research them ourselves, or just look at the label in the grocery store. It's a good idea to start thinking in terms of calories. Try to be as aware of the approximate calories in your next meal as you are of the money in your bank account or the price of a gallon of gas before you put it into your car. It's a great first step to knowing that you're not overeating.

Carbs: Going brown

Carbohydrates are the most basic primary energy source for our bodies, and are broken straight down into glucose. Carbohydrates can either be simple—such as sugary foods—or complex, such as whole-grain breads, potatoes and whole-wheat pasta. The National Institutes of Health (NIH) recommends that about 40 to 60 percent of our total energy intake be from carbohydrates, and primarily the complex kind. The fad, especially among certain dieters in recent years, has been to cut down heavily on carbohydrate intake and increase consumption of other nutrients such as proteins. This is the basis of the famous Atkins diet on which many people have reported significant weight loss (more about that later too). The fact remains, however, that carbohydrates are an important energy source, and if we cut down too heavily on these, then we have to rely on other sources instead, whether they are proteins or fats.

Not all carbohydrates are created equal. The effect of any given carbohydrate on our blood glucose levels is measured using a scale known as the *glycemic index*. High-glycemic index foods, such as cookies, doughnuts, white bread and potatoes produce sharp rises in blood sugar after we eat them. These foods tend to be the worst for us. The second concept we should consider is known as the *glycemic load*. This takes into account the total quantity of carbohydrate consumed as well as the glycemic index. In general, the more fiber a carbohydrate contains, the lower both its glycemic index and glycemic load, and the better it is for us. One large study from Harvard University followed more than 75,000 initially healthy, middle-aged women for a decade and found that those women who regularly consumed carbohydrates with the highest glycemic loads had a staggering *98 percent higher* risk of heart disease when compared to those with the lowest intakes.[3] This was after adjusting for typical coronary risk factors and age.

Among the most unfavorable carbohydrates are those made of white flour. Did you know, for example, that white bread is only white because of a refining process that removes all traces of the bran, or husk, layer? This is actually the main part of the grain that is good for us, containing most of the fiber. It has been estimated that processing whole grains into white flour reduces fiber content by up to 80 percent and increases calories by 10 percent. Refined grains also have a lower water content, which further contributes to the higher calorie count. If that doesn't sound bad enough, the bread is then often turned white by a process involving chemical bleaching agents. So every time you eat a sandwich, pizza, or a hamburger bun that is made with white flour, remember that the refining process has removed most of the good nutrients from what you are eating, as well as often adding chemical bleach! Multiple studies have confirmed the drawbacks of regularly consuming white bread. One study from Melbourne, Australia, involved close to 37,000 people between the ages of 40 and 70.[4] The participants were all given a food frequency questionnaire that assessed their dietary habits, and were followed for four years. By the end of the study, it was found that the odds of getting diabetes were *37 percent higher* in the group that ate the most white bread, compared to those who ate the least. The researchers concluded that switching from white bread to other breads with lower-glycemic indexes, such as brown or whole-grain, could significantly reduce diabetes risk. Other research has even shown that the benefits of switching from refined grains to whole grains may even occur much more quickly. A team from Scotland, for example, recruited more than 200 people and divided them into three groups; each group ate different amounts of whole-grain foods.[5] After only 12 weeks, the groups that increased their whole-grain intake were found to have significantly lower blood pressures. As the medical community knows, high blood pressure is one of the leading causes of heart attacks and strokes. The authors calculated that if this result were repeated across the whole population, there would be a *15 percent decrease* in heart disease, and *25 percent decrease* in strokes.

This negative effect of refining applies equally to rice. In another large investigation, researchers looked at the association between white and brown rice consumption and risk of diabetes.[6]

Almost 40,000 men and 160,000 women were followed for more than 20 years, being given food questionnaires every four years to check on their nutrition habits. By the end of the study, it was found that people who reported the highest intakes of white rice, greater than five servings a week, had a *17 percent increased risk* of diabetes compared to those who consumed it less than once a week. In total contrast, brown rice was associated with an *11 percent decreased risk* of diabetes in those who consumed it the most.

Unfortunately, I rarely see brown rice served in restaurants. Sometimes I even get a quizzical look from the server when I ask! You may be asking, if whole grains are this good for us, how did we get to the point where we are so dependent on refined grains? The answer, unsurprisingly, lies mainly with cost. Refined carbohydrates are easily mass-produced as a carbohydrate-dense economical food, and since the 1960s our intake of refined carbohydrates has been steadily increasing. But the message from scientists couldn't be any clearer: When you consume carbohydrates, go for the carbs that are high in fiber and have a lower glycemic index and load. See the list at the end of this chapter for more examples. Always go brown wherever possible and increase your whole-grain intake to improve your cardiovascular risk. Next time you are in the sandwich or bagel shop and the server asks you which bread you want, choose whole-wheat or whole-grain bread. And what if you already have high-risk conditions such as diabetes or heart disease? Remember, it's never too late to change your habits. Studies have shown that people who have switched from a high to a low-gycemic index diet can experience quick improvements in their disease state.[7]

Many of these medical benefits are directly linked to the increased fiber content in brown carbohydrates. The word itself comes from the Latin word *fibra,* which means thread or string. It is also known as roughage. Fiber is made of non-starch polysaccharides, such as cellulose, and is the indigestible part of plant foods that pushes its way through our digestive system, absorbing water along the way. In addition to the cardiovascular advantages you've just read about, research has shown that people who eat high-fiber diets have reduced rates of cancer, especially of the colon.[8,9] Other studies have shown lower rates of breast and prostate cancers.[10,11] Because it reduces the glycemic load, high- fiber food also slows the spike in glucose we get after eating. Best of all though, fiber actually has *zero* calories and its bulk will leave you feeling full faster. The recommended daily fiber intake is at least 35 grams for men and 25 grams for women. One slice of whole-wheat bread will contain about 3 to 4 grams, a cup of oatmeal 5 grams, an apple 4 ½ grams, and a bowl of black beans 15 grams. Yet despite all the great health effects of fiber, statistics show that we don't eat anywhere near enough of it. Disappointingly, the average American consumes only 10 to 15 grams a day.[12]

Protein: Going white

Protein is needed throughout our body. We get it primarily from meat and dairy products. The amount you need every day depends on your size and weight, and again there are many online calculators that can help you work out how much protein you should be eating. I'm a vegetarian, so I can't speak for myself, but if we're talking about meat, the most important difference to bear in mind is between white and red meat. In health and well-being terms, they are like *chalk and cheese*. White meat includes chicken, poultry and fish. Red meat includes beef, lamb and pork. As well as being high in saturated fats, consuming a lot of red meat has a number of proven harmful effects. A massive study conducted by the National Cancer Institute (NCI) explored the relationship of different types of meat to mortality.[13] Approximately half a million middle-aged people were studied from across the United States, and all answered food questionnaires which assessed their meat intake. The participants were then followed for a decade. By the end of the study, the researchers found some startling and worrying trends. Men and women who reported higher intakes of red and processed meat all clearly had higher mortality risk. Specifically, cancer mortality increased by *22 percent* and cardiovascular risk by *50 percent*. These are huge percentages. As with most research studies, mathematical models were used to correct for confounding variables such as smoking and other lifestyle differences. Interestingly, when the researchers looked at white meat intake and health risk, there was actually an *inverse* association. In other words, the people with the highest intake of white meat did much better than those with the lowest intakes.

A big news story in recent years has been the association between red meat and colon cancer, and the evidence is certainly out there to support this link. One study published in the *Journal of the American Medical Association* looked at the relationship between long-term meat consumption and risk of colon cancer.[14] Almost 150,000 middle-aged adults were studied from across America using a large database which included self-reported dietary habits. The results showed that high intake of red and processed meat led to a higher risk of colon cancer, up to *50 percent* in some cases. Again, on the other side of the coin, this association did not exist with fish and poultry consumption. This finding was backed up by a large investigation from Europe that showed a similar trend in almost half a million men and women from 10 European countries who were followed for five years.[15] Here, the rate of colon cancer increased by *35 percent* with higher red and processed meat intake, but was inversely associated with fish intake.

These results may apply to other cancers as well. Another NIH team studied more than 52,000 middle-aged women for more than five years and found a *23 percent increased* rate of breast cancer when comparing the highest to the lowest self-reported intakes.[16] Finally, as if this isn't enough, a study from Australia of more than 6,700 people even found an almost *50 percent increased* odds of developing macular degeneration, a leading cause of blindness, with higher red meat intake.[17]

You probably get the message by now. Red meat is not the best thing to be eating regularly. And why all these negative outcomes? Scientists are still debating the exact cellular mechanisms involved. One theory is that red meat could contain higher levels of carcinogens (cancer-causing compounds) as well as other substances that increase oxidative damage to cells. Another fact is that red meats are high in saturated fat, which we will come to shortly.

Apart from meat, there are many other great sources of protein too—including dairy products. An average egg, for example, contains about 6.5 grams of protein, most of which is in the egg white. Being vegetarian, I am a big fan of soy protein. Soybeans are the only common plant food that contain complete protein—including all of the amino acids. Soybeans are also a rich source of calcium, iron, B-vitamins and fiber. Soy can be found in tofu, soy milk and tempeh. A large body of evidence supports the beneficial effects of consuming soy protein, and a study published in the prestigious *New England Journal of Medicine* showed that people who consumed soy at an average of 47 grams per day achieved impressive improvements in cholesterol levels of almost *13 percent*.[18] In response to this and other studies, in 1999 the US Food and Drug Administration (FDA) approved claims on product labels that soy helps to reduce heart-related diseases.

So the most important take-home message when it comes to protein is to cut down on red meat and to replace it with other more healthy protein sources such as white meat, soy and low-fat dairy products.

Fats: Not always bad

Okay, here comes the dreaded word. *Fats*. Common wisdom would tell us that there is little to be gained from consuming these.

Well, to an extent yes; for the most part, fats aren't good for us and we should try to avoid them as much as possible. But at the same time, we actually do need them in our diet because they form a vital part of our cells and are needed for the absorption of other nutrients such as vitamins. After carbohydrates, fats are the main secondary energy source for our bodies. They are broadly divided into *saturated* and *unsaturated* fats, and here lies the crucial difference. Saturated fats raise the level of low-density lipoprotein (LDL), which is the "bad" cholesterol. They are found in animal products such as fatty meats, butter, cheese and full-fat dairy products. It is this cholesterol build-up that clogs our arteries and leads to vascular problems. Unsaturated fats are better for us, and the evidence suggests that they help increase high-density lipoprotein (HDL), which is the "good" cholesterol, and also help lower the "bad" cholesterol. The *type* of fat is therefore more important than total fat in our diet. The general recommendation has been that total fat should be less than 30 percent of our total energy intake.

Unsaturated fats can be further divided into monounsaturated and polyunsaturated fats, terms which are plastered over many food boxes and cartons these days. Monounsaturated fats are found in olive and canola oils. Polyunsaturated fats are contained in fish, sunflower and soy bean oils. Omega-3 fatty acids are a type of polyunsaturated fatty acid found in fish oils, flaxseed oil and walnuts. In one large review, a team of researchers set about investigating the effect of increasing polyunsaturated fat intake in place of saturated fats, specifically looking at heart disease rates.[19] They analyzed eight major trials, involving more than 13,600 people, and calculated that there was a *10 percent reduced* heart disease risk for every 5 percent increase in energy from polyunsaturated fatty acids. Scientists believe that some of this effect may also be due to cutting out the saturated fats, as opposed to the direct effects of polyunsaturated fats. Nevertheless, the study result was still striking. Other research has linked the consumption of unsaturated fats to lowered risk of Alzheimer's disease and cognitive decline. In one study from Chicago, investigators followed more than 800 older people and used questionnaires to assess the amount and type of fat intake.[20] After four years of follow-up, the people who consumed the most saturated fat were more than *twice as likely* to develop Alzheimer's disease compared with those who had the lowest intake. In contrast, consumption of polyunsaturated fats had an inverse relationship, indicating a protective effect.

You may have also heard the term "trans fats" a lot in the news. The reason they have generated a lot of publicity is that they are one of the worst foods you can possibly eat. Trans fats are formed during a commercial process known as hydrogenation, which involves the hardening of vegetable fatty oils. Not only do they increase the bad LDL cholesterol, research shows that they also lower the good HDL cholesterol.[21] In other words, double trouble, that can rapidly lead to clogging of your arteries. Trans fats are contained in oils that are maintained at high temperatures for a long time, like those used for deep frying in fast food restaurants. You will therefore find them in fries, doughnuts, cookies and other processed manufactured foods. Also, watch how much butter you use. A study from the Heart Foundation of Australia found that butter can have up to *20 times* the amount of trans fats compared to margarine.[22] Avoid adding too much whenever possible, especially when cooking. Margarine is higher in polyunsaturated fats, so is a much healthier option. Look out for the words "partially hydrogenated" on food labels—they are really not much better than fully hydrogenated fats. No studies have ever found any benefits to consuming trans fats, so you're really better off just cutting them out of your diet completely. Fortunately, many jurisdictions and food outlets are in the process of banning them altogether. Research from the University of Minnesota confirmed the responsiveness of fast food chains to this issue. Analyzing French fries from five of the biggest companies in the country, the researchers showed that since the late 1990s, trans fat content has significantly decreased.[23]

From now on then, whenever you buy any products from the store that are likely to contain fats, whether it be dairy products, meats or butter, it's a good idea to take a second to look at the label and ask two simple questions: Number one, is it high in saturated or polyunsaturated fats, and number two, does it contain trans or partially hydrogenated fats? Often you can find alternative healthy brands if you take the time to look. I've encountered many people who buy any brand of butter at the grocery store without even looking at the label. Don't do this. After all, if it's the wrong type of fat it will go straight to your arteries. Another option if you're not consuming enough polyunsaturated fats is to consider taking an omega-3 fish oil supplement every day. We recommend this to many patients who want a more conservative approach to managing their cholesterol levels.

Fruits and vegetables: Not just a bumper sticker

Fruits and vegetables are an abundant source of the vitamins and minerals that our bodies need. Current estimates suggest that less than a third of adults consume fruits two or more times a day, with only around a quarter eating vegetables three or more times per day.[24] That is shocking. Globally, the problem is even greater. The World Health Organization (WHO) estimates that up to 2.7 million lives could be saved annually with sufficient fruit and vegetable intake.

In response to these abysmal numbers, the Centers for Disease Control and Prevention (CDC) started a campaign resulting in new recommendations based on "cups" rather than "servings" per day, designed to make it easier for us to visualize (the previous recommendation was for at least five servings per day). Now, the exact number of cups is based on our age, gender and physical activity levels, and equates to approximately 4 to 7 cups per day, not including potatoes.

Studies consistently back up the wonderful benefits of eating lots of fruits and vegetables. A large review from the United Kingdom calculated that people who consumed the most fruits and vegetables had a *15 percent lower* risk of heart disease compared to those who reported the least intake.[25] Another team gained data from almost 85,000 women and 42,000 men who were followed for eight years as part of two larger research studies, and showed an even more impressive result.[26] This time, people who consumed the highest amounts of fruits and vegetables had a *20 percent decreased* risk compared to those with the least intake. Green leafy vegetables and vitamin C-rich fruits appeared to have the most effect.

Similar dramatic benefits have been found with other conditions too. Stroke, one of the most devastating and debilitating acute medical events, has also been shown to occur less frequently in people who consume the most fruits and vegetables. A study published in the *Journal of the American Medical Association* looked at data from more than 830 middle-aged men who were followed over a 20-year period.[27] When the results were analyzed, it was calculated that for every increase of three servings per day, the risk of stroke *decreased by 22 percent*, and for some types of stroke *more than 50 percent*. Further research has shown reduced rates of diabetes, and inverse associations with chronic disease and tooth decay.[28-30] If statistics like these aren't a reason to order that extra salad, then nothing will be!

So what is it about fruits and vegetables that produces such astonishing benefits? The most obvious theory is that the natural substances they contain, like vitamins, minerals and potassium, exert a directly positive effect on our cells that results in outcomes like improved immunity, cell repair and lower blood pressure. Another theory is that as we eat *more* fruits and vegetables, we eat *less* of the bad foods, such as candies and chips. Counteracting this, however, is the fact that many of the studies take into account other dietary intake in their statistical analyses, and correct for this, but still show the same benefits.

Fruits and vegetables are also a prime source of substances that have become a buzzword in recent years: *Antioxidants*. Antioxidants protect your cells against the effects of free radicals, which are molecules produced when your body burns oxygen. Free radicals damage cells, and have been shown to play important roles in aging, cancer and heart disease. Natural antioxidants include Vitamins A, C, E and Beta-carotene. In general, the darker and more colored any fruit or vegetable is, such as berries or pomegranates, the more likely it is to be high in antioxidants. Consuming more of these is recommended, but so far additional supplementation with pills has yet to be proven in scientific studies. Bear in mind, too, that antioxidants are not found only in fruits and vegetables per se. Tea, especially green tea, also has a high antioxidant content, and is probably one of the healthiest drinks out there (tea does, of course, initially come from leaves, so maybe we are justified in thinking of it as an honorary vegetable).

A final major benefit of fruits and vegetables is that they are relatively low in calories and leave us feeling full, so they're a great part of any weight management strategy. We have so many choices right there in front of us as soon as we enter the grocery store. It's helpful that fruits and vegetables are often the first section as we walk through the door. Apples, blueberries, oranges, bananas, pears, kiwis, strawberries, lettuce, broccoli, spinach, cucumbers, tomatoes, carrots and onions. Don't walk past them next time without placing loads of them in your cart! If your favorite fruit or vegetable is out of season, you can also buy the frozen kind and still get many of the benefits (just don't buy the ones frozen in sugary syrup).

Apples and Blueberries: Two special fruits

The apple tree was one of the earliest trees to be cultivated, and is widely depicted in ancient mythology. Today, there are more than 7,500 known varieties of apple, so there are plenty to choose from. The age-old saying that *an apple a day keeps the doctor away* is not just an old wives' tale. It's actually backed up by solid research. In an article entitled, "Does an apple a day keep the oncologist away?,"' researchers in Milan, Italy, conducted a review of several larger studies.[31] In total, data were collected from almost 600 patients who were divided into two groups according to self-reported apple consumption of either less than one per day, or one or more apples a day. This revealed a strong *inverse* relationship for all types of cancers studied, including oral, esophagus, colon, breast, ovary and prostate. Even when other factors were corrected for, such as overall consumption of fruits and vegetables, this association persisted. The study concluded that the beneficial effects of eating apples was potentially linked to the *catechins* and *flavonol* antioxidants that they contain. A fascinating piece of research from Cornell University involved a laboratory investigation where a group of rats with a known genetic predisposition to breast cancer was fed apple extracts.[32] The results showed that the number of tumors, when compared to a control group of similar rats not fed apple extracts, was reduced by a staggering *25 to 61 percent* in rats that were fed the human equivalent of one to six apples a day. The researchers again put this effect down to the *phytochemical* antioxidants in apples. Obviously, we can't eat six apples a day, and humans are different from rats (hopefully, most of the time anyway), but the dramatic reduction in tumors from such a simple intervention was truly an amazing finding. One further experiment from the same university points to a direct benefit for our brain too. This time, the team of scientists successfully demonstrated that apple nutrients provided a protective effect for brain neurons against the oxidative damage that can trigger diseases like Alzheimer's and Parkinson's. Their experiments showed a massive *70 to 90 percent reduction* in accumulated reactive oxygen species in neurons exposed to apple nutrients such as quercetins.[33]

The list goes on and on, with other studies revealing benefits for cholesterol build-up, asthma, lung function, and even lessened allergy symptoms in children whose mothers consumed more apples during pregnancy![34-37] In addition, remember that apples are also high in fiber, of which we've already seen the advantages. This is yet another time when your mom was indeed right. An apple a day really does help keep the doctor away. And how many apples do we each consume in a *week*? On average, only *one*. That's a big missed opportunity for a tasty and widely available fruit to improve our health.

If apples are this good, then blueberries may be even better. They have one of the highest known antioxidant contents of any food, in the form of compounds known as *polyphenols* and *anthocyanins*, which are responsible for the blue pigment. In fact, 100 grams of fresh blueberries can contain more antioxidant properties than five whole servings of fruits and vegetables. When the US Department of Agriculture (USDA) laboratory in Boston ranks foods according to antioxidant activity, blueberries consistently rank near the top of the list, followed by cranberries, strawberries, raspberries and artichokes.

Scientific studies back up the terrific effects of eating blueberries. In one study from Greece, researchers injected a group of mice with polyphenol extracts from wild blueberries every day for one week.[38] When they were tested afterwards with specially designed tasks to evaluate their learning and memory functions, the mice that were given the highest amounts of blueberry extracts showed significantly better performance in both of these parameters. They also had direct evidence of higher brain antioxidant activity. A second experiment, also conducted in mice (and hopefully by now you can see why such direct brain experiments would be difficult to conduct in humans!) showed that polyphenols from blueberries promoted a mechanism known as autophagy in brain cells, which is the natural process by which damaged cells are recognized.[39] As animals age, autophagy declines, which can lead to the degeneration involved in memory decline. Consuming berries could, therefore, exert an anti-aging effect.

Reassuringly, positive results have been extended to human research too. An interesting study from the University of Oklahoma investigated the effects of blueberries on cardiovascular risk factors in obese men and women.[40] The researchers took almost 50 participants, mainly female and obese, and gave them either a freeze-dried blueberry drink or an equivalent amount of water to drink every day for eight weeks. The results were amazing for such a low-cost intervention. The women who consumed the blueberry drink had significant drops in their blood pressures after eight weeks when compared to the control group. As for the other major cardiovascular risk factor—diabetes—a team from Louisiana performed another experiment that took 32 obese, non-diabetic people and divided them into two groups.[41] One group received a twice-daily smoothie containing blueberry extract, and the other received a similar smoothie but without the blueberry content. After six weeks, the blueberry group was found to have improved insulin sensitivity, which plays an important role in reducing diabetes risk. Studies like this go to show that even when the beneficial nutrient is contained in a smoothie, which isn't necessarily the healthiest option, there still may be a profoundly positive effect. In the same way, a blueberry muffin will be better than a regular muffin—if you must eat a muffin, that is!

These health effects of blueberries also likely apply to some of their cousins too. Bear in mind that strawberries, raspberries and blackberries all contain similar chemical compounds and antioxidants, albeit slightly less. We are unlikely to get large-scale scientific studies that investigate each and every one, but all the evidence clearly points in one direction—berries are extremely good for us. So make a deliberate effort to improve both your blueberry and apple intake. If you don't find them tasty alone, then be creative and add them to another dish (toss a handful of blueberries in to your oatmeal or a salad, for example, or bake an apple and add a sprinkling of cinnamon to spice it up). However you like these powerhouse fruits, make sure you get your fill.

Some nutty evidence

There has been much controversy in recent years regarding the health benefits of nuts. Are they good for us or not? I remember hearing over the years that eating nuts is unhealthy because they are high in calories and fat. While this is true, remember what we said about not all fats being bad. The latest research actually suggests that most nuts, especially walnuts and almonds, are an excellent source of unsaturated fats, particularly omega-3 fatty acids. Therefore, nuts can be good for us and help to lower our bad cholesterol. A study from Loma Linda University investigated the effects of nuts by gathering data from 25 nut-consumption trials involving more than 580 people in seven countries.[42] The results yielded a dramatic result. Daily consumption of 67 grams, or approximately one handful, of nuts achieved a *5 percent reduction* in total cholesterol, *7.5 percent reduction* in the bad LDL cholesterol, and *10 percent reduction* in triglycerides. Better still, the researchers found that different types of nuts all had similar effects and that the benefits were most pronounced among those who already had high cholesterol and who consumed Western diets. Another large review, this one looking specifically at walnuts, combined results from several smaller studies, and calculated that diets supplemented by walnuts resulted in an approximately *10 point decrease* in total and LDL cholesterol levels, while having no adverse effect on weight.[43]

According to USDA statistics, 100 grams of walnuts contain approximately 15 grams of protein, 7 grams of fiber and 65 grams of fat, of which almost 75 percent are healthy polyunsaturated fatty acids. In 2004 the FDA approved the claim that "eating 1.5 oz of walnuts per day, about 10 walnuts, as part of a low saturated fat and low cholesterol diet, and not resulting in increased caloric intake, may reduce the risk of coronary heart disease."

If you don't like walnuts, evidence shows that almonds can have an impressive effect on cholesterol levels too.[44] Brazil and pecan nuts are likely not too far behind either. As long as you have no allergies or intolerances, start eating more nuts from now on. But do keep in mind that nuts also have a relatively high calorie count, so if you start eating them regularly, cut something else out of your diet to make up for this.

Just a pinch of salt

Salt is a scourge of today's society. We eat way too much of it, which results in our bodies retaining excess water, putting us at increased risk of conditions like high blood pressure and heart disease. The recommended daily allowance of sodium is 2,300 milligrams, or approximately *one teaspoon a day*. People at high risk for heart disease, like those with diabetes or a strong family history, should be consuming less than 1,500 milligrams per day. Despite these recommendations, government statistics reveal that the average daily salt consumption stands at over 3,400 milligrams! It isn't surprising, then, that an analysis published in the *New England Journal of Medicine* concluded that modest reductions in salt intake in the population could result in massive improvements in heart disease and stroke rates, and also be more cost-effective than using expensive medications to reduce blood pressure.[45] Be especially careful with processed or packaged foods, which tend to contain pure sodium as opposed to the sodium chloride in our table salt. It is not uncommon for a can of soup to contain more than 1,000 milligrams of salt, and two sausages can contain almost 2,500 milligrams—more than your whole daily allowance. Also, try not to add too much when you cook. Generally, when it comes to salt, the less, the better.

Going vegetarian

As a vegetarian, I may be biased when I say this, but the potential health benefits of cutting down on meat are enormous. We've already seen the harmful effects of eating too much red meat. Going vegetarian is also great for the planet because it cuts down on the associated environmental pressures involved in raising livestock. It has been estimated that 20 percent of all greenhouse emissions are from animal farming!

Research has linked vegetarian diets to improved diabetes control, lower cancer rates, reduced childhood obesity, and even higher IQ.[46-49] In a large investigation, data were tracked on almost 130,000 people for more than two decades, all of whom were on either self-reported vegetable-based or meat-based diets.[50] The results found that people who reported more meat-based diets had a *23 percent higher* mortality rate, *14 percent higher* cardiovascular mortality and *28 percent higher* cancer mortality. On the other hand, a higher vegetable-based diet was associated with a *20 percent decreased* mortality rate and *23 percent lower* cardiovascular mortality.

Consider having a dedicated day every week when you don't eat meat. If you can do it two days, even better. By vegetarian, we are only talking about meat intake. I am not advocating a vegan diet, which doesn't allow dairy products like milk and cheese, or eggs, all of which are good sources of the protein you need.

Chocolate

I love to eat chocolate. I blame my mom for that, as she loves her sweets too. My dad is the opposite, and doesn't find himself at all drawn to sugary foods. You either have a sweet tooth or you don't. The majority of us do however! Chocolate is relatively high in simple carbohydrates and saturated fats, so nutritional science would hold that chocolate is something to be avoided. I'm going to tell you something very different. You don't necessarily need to cut chocolate completely out of your diet. Treating yourself is fine, and in fact, may even be *beneficial* to your health.

A team of researchers from Sweden followed more than 1,100 people who had suffered a heart attack.[51] They asked all of the participants to fill out questionnaires about their chocolate consumption. Now you would expect that those eating the most chocolate would have the worst outcomes—right? *Wrong*. Chocolate consumption had a strong *inverse* association with cardiovascular mortality over an eight-year period. Compared with those who never ate chocolate, people who ate it up to once a week had a *44 percent lower* mortality rate, and those who were even more mischievous, and admitted eating chocolate twice or more a week had a staggering *66 percent lower* rate. When the data was analyzed further, there was no relationship with other types of candy. This finding was not an anomaly. In another study, researchers followed more than 1,200 older Australian women for almost a decade.[52] Again, they found that those who consumed chocolate more than once a week were almost *25 percent less likely* to be hospitalized for vascular complications and *35 percent less likely* to develop heart disease, when compared to rare chocolate eaters.

Can it really be true, for a nice change, that something so naughty can be good for us? And if so, what causes this? Scientists believe that some of these benefits are mediated by the bioactive compounds, such as *flavonoids*, found in cocoa. There may also be a difference between the chocolates in different countries too, with European dark chocolates believed to be better. Unfortunately, none of this means that you should gorge yourself with chocolate in the interests of your health (sorry, everyone). It's especially not a good idea if you are dieting, which we will come to soon. But it does show that eating a small amount—1 to 2 ounces per serving—a few times a week is not only okay, but may even be good for you.

Going Mediterranean

When it comes to healthy eating, we can learn a lot from some other parts of the world. Two areas in particular that are known for their outstanding dietary habits are the *Mediterranean* and *Japan*. Without meaning to neglect the Japanese diet, which actually has many similarities to that eaten in the Mediterranean, Japanese food is probably not something most of us can fit into our schedule and budget on a daily basis, so we will leave that for another time and place.

The benefits of adopting a Mediterranean diet have been well portrayed in the media. In a nutshell, this involves generous portions of fruits and vegetables, more whole grains, healthy fats like olive and canola oil, very little red meat (instead replacing it with seafood), and spices and herbs rather than salt to flavor food. Mediterraneans also regularly eat small portions of nuts, and drink low to moderate amounts of red wine. And away from eating, they are known for sitting down to enjoy meals with their family and friends, and also for getting plenty of exercise. It's a whole way of life that revolves around healthy nutrition. As a result of these admirable habits, people in countries like Italy and Spain have some of the best health statistics in the world, and can be expected to be physically fit and free of illness well into old age. Anybody who has worked in healthcare and has dealt with people of Mediterranean descent already knows how healthy (and family-oriented) many of them are.

Research has time and again backed up the advantages of a Mediterranean diet in terms of cardiovascular risk, longevity and even cognitive decline. One massive review from Italy that analyzed results from a dozen other published studies, involving a mind-blowing 1.5 million people who were followed for up to 18 years, showed that increased adherence to the diet was associated with an almost *10 percent reduced* mortality risk, *6 percent lower* cancer rates and *13 percent lower* risk of Parkinson's disease and Alzheimer's dementia.[53] It is obvious from results like this that Mediterranean people are doing something incredibly right that we in other Western countries are not. As if to reinforce this point, and our own fallibility, the evidence shows that when Mediterranean people move from their own countries to other Western nations, their health statistics often quickly fall in line with our countries as they adopt the bad habits of their new homeland.

A saying we have in the medical field goes that *heart disease rates are low where the olive tree grows*. At the most fundamental level, a Mediterranean diet follows the same basic rules for carbohydrate, protein, healthy fats and fruit and vegetable intake that we have just gone over in this chapter. They are maximizing their wellness through their diet, and it's worth our emulating their behaviors.

Start healthier eating

In this chapter, we have gone over some of the basic nutrition steps that can result in significant health benefits. The scientific evidence for eating complex carbs, cutting back on red meat, consuming healthy fats and increasing your fruit and vegetable intake is compelling and unquestionable. Wasn't a lot of it just common knowledge anyway? We already knew that there is a problem with overeating in society. We've already heard that fatty foods are bad, and have been told countless times to eat more whole-wheat bread and finish our greens. But now you've seen the solid medical testimony too. Obviously, as with anything in life, exercise your own sensible judgment as well. If you start eating kilos of brown bread, walnuts or olive oil, then that's not a good thing either! Moderation rules the day. Even the healthiest foods in the world may have some drawbacks. An apple, for example, still contains some simple carbohydrates, and olive oil still contains a bit of saturated fat. But take on board all of the points and try to implement at least some of them next time you plan a meal or go grocery shopping.

Remember that eating habits are about more than just the actual food. How we eat, including the size of our plates and where we dine, can also have a large impact. For instance, people tend to eat more food when they're in front of the television than they would sitting at the dinner table. Unfortunately, statistics show that dining with the family is becoming more rare. Having regular sit-down meals used to be the typical evening routine for every American family. Family dining time also has positive social implications too; one study from Columbia University revealed that children who regularly ate dinner with their families were less likely to smoke, drink or use drugs.[54] Try to promote a regular sit-down meal with your family every day and you'll all reap the rewards in so many ways.

Small steps count. There's always something you can do to make your next meal a little bit healthier. Load your sandwich with greens. Make sure at least half your plate is filled with vegetables. Order only whole-grain bagels. Even if you have a less-than-healthy meal, you can always make it healthier. Have a thin-crust pizza instead of deep dish, or top your dish of ice cream with fresh fruit! One of my own favorite desserts is to mix walnuts and blueberries into some low-fat yogurt. If you start with small changes, they will all eventually add up.

Don't be too hard on yourself either. You don't have to become overly restrictive or obsessive. Treats are totally okay—indeed, life would be boring if you didn't allow yourself any indulgences every now and again. But be careful that *treat* doesn't become *habit*. You can set yourself a limit, such as eating only a limited number of desserts or take-outs a week. Adopting a healthier eating plan is fun and rewarding. In today's world, you are spoiled for choice and have a wealth of options. Your good eating habits will likely spread to those around you—family, friends and colleagues. It's actually much more difficult to *stop* caring about your diet once you begin. So start making those changes right away and the benefits will be there at your fingertips.

HIGH PERCENTAGE NUTRITION WELLNESS STEPS

- Start thinking in terms of calories

    Know the approximate amounts in your next meal or snack

- Consume non-refined, brown carbohydrates

    Whole-wheat and whole-grain products and brown rice are good choices

- Increase your fiber intake

    Choose high-fiber bread, cereals, oatmeal, beans and lentils

- Cut down on red meat

    Get your protein from white meat, eggs, dairy products and soy

- Replace saturated with polyunsaturated fats

    Use vegetable and fish oils, and margarine instead of butter

- Eat fruits and vegetables at every opportunity

    Add multiple portions every day, with every meal

- Enjoy apples and blueberries at least once a day

    Make this a regular habit

- Consume healthy portions of nuts

    Walnuts and almonds are great choices

- Beware of hidden salt

    Avoid processed foods and don't add too much when you cook

- Go vegetarian

    Skip meat at least 1-2 days a week

- Live like the Mediterraneans

    Copy their healthy eating habits

NATURAL ANTIOXIDANTS

- **Vitamin A and Beta-carotene**

    Choose colorful fruits and vegetables such as carrots, spinach, apricots, mangos, broccoli

- **Vitamin C**

    Enjoy citrus fruits, tomatoes, strawberries, broccoli, red and green peppers

- **Vitamin E**

    Almonds, walnuts, sunflower seeds and wheat germ oil

- **Phenols**

    Eat berries, apples, grapes and citrus fruits

GLYCEMIC INDEX LIST

High glycemic index (greater than 70)

Cut down on white bread, baguettes, white rice, potatoes, French fries and doughnuts

Medium glycemic index (56-69)

Add whole-wheat bread and brown rice on a moderate basis

Low glycemic index (less than 55)

Enjoy whole and multi-grain bread, oatmeal, all-bran, beans, legumes, lentils, most fruits and vegetables

Approximate examples, exact values vary by product and method of cooking. Please only consume foods based on your own dietary requirements and medical history, based on advice from your own physician. Certain fruits may not be regularly advisable in diabetes, and nuts should be eaten with caution by anyone with a history of nut allergy or intolerance

CHAPTER TWO

ACTIVITY WELLNESS:
THE INCREDIBLE BENEFITS OF EXERCISE

Sometime in the last 50 years we have become a society of couch potatoes. Unlike a few decades ago when we were much more active, we now have ample opportunities to avoid getting up, whether we're sitting in front of the television or on the computer. We spend too much time in our cars and drive even the shortest of distances. We have a drive-thru for picking up our fast food and a drive-thru for withdrawing money. Think back over the last week to all the times you avoided walking. Did you hop into the car to drive only a couple of blocks or go from one end of the mall to another, when you could just as easily have taken a quick walk? Did you take the elevator to go up just one floor? There are only a few short steps (literally) that are needed to reverse these habits, but as with diet and nutrition, simple awareness of all the benefits and missed opportunities is the first step. Physical activity and exercise can be one of the most enjoyable, rewarding and personally satisfying experiences you can engage in. Most of us do not get anywhere near enough of it. It can come in many forms—a brisk walk, climbing stairs, running, playing sports or even dancing! While I have heard many people moan about how dull healthy eating feels to them, I've yet to hear anyone say the same thing about exercise. Getting involved in playing sports can be a terrific amount of fun that we can all enjoy in some format. So if it's so great, how come we don't do more of it?

According to the CDC, almost one-third to one-half of all Americans do not meet the minimum goals for exercising, and almost a quarter report absolutely *no* leisure time activity. At the same time, it's estimated that we manage to spend an average of 4 to 5 hours a day watching television. Many people list "not having enough time" as the main reason for not fitting exercise into their daily regimen. If you watch anything more than 30 minutes of television a day, then you probably do have enough time!

What is the difference between physical activity and exercise? They both involve a similar process, but their strict definitions are somewhat different. Physical activity is anything that increases your resting energy requirements. It can mean something as simple as climbing the stairs or running to catch the train. Exercise, on the other hand, is defined as bodily exertion, typically in an organized fashion, such as jogging or playing a sport.

When you exert yourself, a number of physiological changes occur within your body. Your heart rate and blood pressure increase, leading to more blood being pumped through your arteries, and consequently, more oxygen being delivered to your cells. This happens even when you are climbing the stairs or running to catch that train. Your blood vessels dilate and your respiratory system responds by trying to take in more oxygen, hence making you feel short of breath. When you undertake sustained activity such as exercise, these changes occur for a prolonged period as your body works to provide energy for all of your working muscles. More blood is getting to your brain as well, which produces many other desirable effects. First and foremost though, we are exerting the heart muscle, as it works to keep up with the body's demands.

How much we need

The current recommendation from the CDC is for the following amount of activity each week:

• Two-and-a-half hours (150 minutes) of moderate-intensity aerobic activity, or

• One-and-a-quarter hours (75 minutes) of vigorous-intensity aerobic activity

This is based on recommendations from both the American Heart Association and the American College of Sports Medicine, which states that "to promote and maintain health, all healthy adults aged 18 to 65 need moderate-intensity physical activity for a minimum of 30 minutes on five days each week, or vigorous-intensity aerobic physical activity for a minimum of 20 minutes on three days each week." Even in old age, these recommendations still apply as long as you are healthy enough. Moderate-intensity activity is something like brisk walking, while vigorous activity is running or playing a sport intensely. In addition, it is also recommended that every adult perform muscle-strengthening exercises at least two days per week. You don't have to be an Arnold Schwarzenegger, but as your regular muscle fibers build up in your arms and legs, the same is believed to happen with your heart muscle, making it stronger too. A study of almost 8,800 men in Sweden between the ages of 20 and 80 found that during an almost 20-year follow-up, those with higher muscle strength had lower mortality rates compared to those with less.[1] So at the very least, add gentle weight exercises with dumbbells or weight machines to your fitness routine to build up your strength.

If 150 minutes a week sounds like a lot, see if you are spending excess time doing other less urgent activities. Divided over the course of a week, that's really not that much time if you do it in 30-minute increments. You can even break it up into much smaller chunks of time during the day. Bouts of activity, such as 10 minutes at a time, are fine and combinations of moderate and vigorous activity can be used to meet this goal. For example, you can go for brisk walks on some days and cycle on others. However you do it, the recommendations should be drilled into your head: 150 minutes of moderate- and 75 minutes of vigorous-intensity aerobic activity.

Over the years, I've met so many patients—not to mention family and friends—who have told me that they exercise just by walking around a lot. As you can see from the recommendations, only *brisk* walking counts as cardiovascular activity. Simple walking is not classified as exercise at all. Physiologically, while it is obviously better than just sitting still, if you are otherwise healthy, walking really doesn't get you up to an optimal cardiovascular level, especially when you are walking casually and on a flat surface. If you want to walk your way to health benefits, walk fast with good arm strides. When you finish, you should feel that you have exerted yourself and experience some breathlessness, fatigue and even sweating. If you feel these symptoms after just casual walking, then you either have an underlying health problem, or you are incredibly unfit!

Keep in mind that these are just *minimal* requirements. As with anything in life, you don't necessarily have to settle for the minimum. The more you are able to surpass these recommendations, the more likely you are to experience the positive effects. Always check with your physician though before introducing any major changes to your exercise regimen, but as long as you are deemed healthy enough, then go for it.

Cardiovascular benefits

The reason why so many authorities advocate regular exercise are the enormous health advantages that have been proven time and again by medical research. It's an understatement to say that the benefits to your cardiovascular system are potentially huge. In one Harvard study, a team of researchers followed almost 45,000 men for 12 years.[2] During this time, approximately 1,700 new cases of heart disease were diagnosed. Using data from regular health checks and completed questionnaires, their results showed that heart disease rates decreased substantially as physical activity levels increased. Overall, those who exercised most frequently had a *30 percent lower* risk of heart disease. Men who reported running for an hour or more per week had a *42 percent risk reduction* compared to those who didn't run. Men who said they walked briskly for half an hour a day had an *18 percent reduction*. A second analysis from Norway yielded even more impressive results, with an almost *60 percent lower* risk of cardiovascular disease in men with the highest levels of physical fitness.[3] Similar results apply to women too, although cardiovascular health studies have traditionally focused more on men than on women—fortunately, that is now changing. An investigation published in the *New England Journal of Medicine* that followed more than 72,000 middle-aged women from the Nurses' Health Study found exactly the same pattern.[4] As the women became more active, their risk of suffering a heart attack decreased by *23 to 54 percent* according to energy expenditure. Those who walked briskly for three or more hours a week had a *35 percent lower risk* compared to those who walked the least. Other large studies have found similarly dramatic results in women—even after correcting for smoking status, alcohol use, diet and family history.[5]

Starting a new exercise routine

If it has never been part of your schedule, you may ask yourself what benefits starting to exercise can now bring you. The answer, like with changing your diet—is many! It's never too late to start exercising, and as long as your doctor gives you the go-ahead, you shouldn't be afraid to get going. A team from Stanford University who analyzed data from almost 10,300 middle-aged and older males for more than eight years found that those who began undertaking moderately vigorous activity had an over *40 percent reduced risk* of cardiovascular mortality and *23 percent lower* mortality compared to those who didn't do the same.[6] Even if you are unfortunate enough to have become sick, exercise can still be extremely beneficial to you. Another group of researchers spent seven years investigating more than 400 people who had recently suffered a heart attack.[7] By the end of the study, their results showed that the people who reported increasing their activity levels had an incredible *90 percent increased* survival rate compared to the most sedentary group. The same people also had an almost *80 percent lower* risk of a repeat heart attack.

You don't even have to perform overly strenuous exercises, especially if you have suffered a recent medical problem. It's understandable in that case if you are anxious about pushing yourself too hard. Just doing something relatively light like gardening, which involves simple stretching exercises, has been found in studies to improve mortality risk and blood pressure.[8,9] Something is always better than nothing.

The benefits apply at any age

The recommendations for physical activity hold forth no matter what your age, as long as your body is able to do so. Obviously an 80-year-old is unlikely to be able to play basketball or run a marathon like a 20-year-old, and it's up to everyone to judge just how far he or she can go. One study from the University of Virginia looked specifically into the effects of walking in older men in their 70s, 80s and even 90s, who lived in Hawaii (a nice place to do an exercise experiment).[10] Data on more than 2,600 men was collected for four years, and when heart disease rates were correlated with reported activity levels, researchers found that men who walked less than a quarter of a mile a day were more than *twice as likely* to get heart disease compared to those who walked more than one-and-a-half miles per day. Every half-mile increase in walking per day resulted in a *15 percent reduced* risk. Further analysis of several hundred men from the same study also confirmed a strong relationship between average distance walked and longevity.[11] Men who walked less than one mile per day had nearly *twice* the mortality rate during the follow-up when compared to those who walked more than two miles per day. And remember, these were men in their 70s, 80s and 90s.

If you're older, the benefits of being active are even more important for you. Get out as much as possible. If you can walk briskly, that's great; otherwise stroll as much as possible. Just like a car that you leave sitting in the garage, you will be prone to problems if you stay stationary. The more you stay active into old age, the better.

At the opposite end of the spectrum, childhood and adolescence has always been the time of life to be the most physically active. This is natural to all animals. Those of us who have had puppies and kittens know how impossible it is to get them to sit still. One unfortunate consequence of the technology revolution is that it unnaturally encourages youngsters to stay sedentary. We will learn shortly what effects this has on obesity, but it really is a great shame what inventions like televisions and video games have done from this point of view. The teenage years are turbulent enough as it is, without lifestyle habits contributing to making things worse! A survey from West Virginia University asked almost 250 teenage middle-school students about their activity levels, self-perception of health and overall life satisfaction.[12] Their answers found that girls who had taken part in vigorous activity in the week prior to the questionnaire experienced significantly higher life satisfaction. In both boys and girls, playing on a sports team was associated with higher life satisfaction. Indeed, girls were 30 *times* more likely, and boys *five times* more likely, to describe their own health as 'fair' or 'poor' if they did not play on a team. This shows that exercising in youth can have dramatic effects at a vital point in development. It's also worth remembering that engaging in sports helps with other skills, such as enhancing social connections and bonding with others.

Other medical benefits

It's not just cardiovascular health that has been found to improve with exercising. Research shows a whole host of other lowered risks too. Another chronic condition that is exploding in prevalence is diabetes. More data analysis from the Nurses' Health Study showed that diabetes risk decreased by *23 to 46 percent* with increasing physical activity.[13] This trend persisted even when the results were adjusted for baseline body mass index (BMI), meaning that the effect of exercise was *independent* of weight. Even walking decreased the risk by up to *42 percent*, especially in the brisk walkers.

Other studies have looked into the relationship between exercise and cancer risk. A team from Dallas followed more than 32,000 middle-aged people and found sharp declines in cancer mortality with increasing physical fitness.[14] The Nurses' Health Study data revealed that women who exercised the most, equivalent to one hour a day of brisk walking, had a *15 percent reduced* breast cancer rate compared to those who were the most sedentary.[15] Even women who increased their activity levels at menopause had a *10 percent reduced* rate compared to those who didn't. And a study result from South Carolina was even more impressive—almost 15,000 women were followed for 16 years, and those with the best fitness levels had a *55 percent lower* breast cancer mortality rate.[16]

Osteoporosis, the bone thinning that occurs in older age which leads to increased fracture risk, can also be partly prevented or delayed by physical activity. This one follows more logic, as obviously the more you use your bones and muscles, the stronger they should become. In one experiment, investigators randomized 160 osteoporotic women over the age of 70 into two groups, one of which performed regular exercise.[17] After following them for seven years, the researchers calculated that the exercise group had a *32 percent reduced* incident rate of new fractures. In fact, the exercise group actually suffered *no* hip fractures. That's a great result.

Exercise during your workday

You may not have thought about this before, but you can actually get quite a lot of exercise during your workday if you try hard enough. Of course, some fields are more strenuous than others. In my line of work as a hospital doctor, I can burn off significant amounts of calories by brisk walking and running up and down stairs. Many other jobs have this potential too. And what about how you get to work? Most of us don't have the opportunity or time to walk or cycle to work, but there are plenty of other things you can do. For example, you don't have to park right next to your office building. Especially if it's a nice day, you can always park a bit further away and walk the rest of the distance. Better still, park on a lower level and take the stairs up to work as well! A study from Finland looked into the effects of job activity levels in more than 3,300 diabetic men and women.[18] Their jobs were categorized as *light* (mainly sitting in a chair), *moderate* (standing and walking more frequently) or *active* (regular manual work such as lifting). Their daily commute was further divided into three categories: motorized transportation with no walking, walking or cycling up to 30 minutes, and walking or cycling for more than 30 minutes (you can see, too, why this type of experiment is easier to do in Finland, because it's practically unheard of for anyone to walk or cycle to work here in America!). During almost 20 years of follow-up, the researchers found that people whose jobs involved *moderate* activity had *20 percent lower* mortality rates, and those that involved *active* work had a *41 percent* improved rate. These calculations corrected for other health problems and physical activity levels outside work, and are even more impressive given that it's usually people in the lower socioeconomic groups who tend to have more physically strenuous occupations and poorer health. With regards to the commute to work, walking and cycling were found to be inversely associated with mortality. For people who had a combination of increased activity in both their commute and in their workplace, the statistics showed a close to *50 percent improved* survival.

Now let's take something simple like taking the stairs. Always relying on elevators represents a huge missed opportunity. During my typical work day, I'm always astounded by the number of very able-bodied staff and visitors (of course, I'm not including the sick patients), who use the elevator to go up or down just one or two levels when the stairs are right next to them. The irony is that for these short trips, it actually takes more than *double* the amount of time just waiting for the elevator than it does to take the stairs! In other words, our own laziness has converted something that was designed to make our lives quicker and easier into something more time-consuming. Sometimes I see people willing to wait several minutes for the elevator instead of just going up the stairs in perhaps

10 or 15 seconds. That's a great shame, because from a purely energy-burning perspective, climbing stairs is a brilliant calorie burner. It's estimated that a person weighing 150 pounds can burn up to 10 calories a minute just by walking up the stairs. Say that your job involves a lot of moving around between different floors, and let's say you weigh 150 pounds and you go up the stairs whenever you can for 30 seconds a time. If you do that 10 times a day, that's already potentially 50 calories burned. For certain jobs like mine, we can take the stairs maybe 20 or 30 times in one day. Imagine all those calories burned. Many employers are realizing that more activity for their employees is a great thing. Some are now even savvy enough to have on-site gyms. Our hospital has a walking track in the foyer to encourage people to walk, and I often see ex-patients coming back to walk around it themselves. Think about your place of work and all the potential exercise you can get in a day.

Exercise for your mood and brain

I'm guessing you've heard before about the mental and emotional effects of exercise. The term *endorphins* is bandied about everywhere these days. But what exactly are they? Endorphins are a type of neurotransmitter, the chemicals in the brain involved in transmitting electrical signals between the billions of neurons. The word "endorphin" actually comes from two words, *endogenous* and *morphine*. There are more than 20 types of endorphins, which are released in significant quantities during exercise, excitement, pain and other activities like eating spicy food. They actually work in a similar fashion to morphine in the way they produce analgesia (pain-relief) and a general feeling of well-being. In exercise circles, this is known as the famous "runner's high." And all physicians and nurses get to see the "morphine high" that patients can experience when we relieve their pain!

Those people who exercise regularly understand what a great feeling it can be to have a good work-out session, followed by a nice shower afterwards. It's a totally natural way to feel good. But just how strong is the scientific evidence for the positive effects of endorphins? Is there a rationale for your doctor to prescribe exercise if you are feeling down? Research from Duke University suggests so.[19] A team of investigators took more than 150 volunteers with a diagnosis of major depression, and divided them randomly into three groups. The first group underwent four months of an exercise program, the second was prescribed a popular antidepressant, and the third was given a combination of both. All of the participants received regular assessments using validated depression scales. The results were thought-provoking. By the end of the study, all groups had experienced a similarly clinically significant reduction in their depression scores. In other words, exercise was *just* as effective as the popular medication for reducing depression symptoms. When these people were followed-up six months later, it was found that participants in the exercise group actually had significantly lower relapse rates than those in the medication group.[20] In the people who exercised on their own after the study finished, there was a *50 percent reduced* risk of depression. The same researchers then conducted a larger study, in more than 200 adults with major depression.[21] This time, one of the groups also received a placebo pill. Like the last study, treatments continued for four months in order to give the medication maximum time to have an effect. Overall, more than *40 percent* of participants achieved remission in their major depression. When comparing the exercise groups to those taking antidepressants, once again, *both* had similar results in terms of curative rates.

In fact, even a short burst of activity can bring about immediate boosts. It's not necessarily a long time before the effects are felt. Another experiment, involving more than 60 volunteers, asked people to perform either an aerobic workout or to just sit and watch a video.[22] Standardized testing revealed a *25 percent increase* in the participants' positive mood after exercise, but a significant *decrease* in mood after video watching. As a bonus, a measure of creativity was found to be significantly higher too. So this is yet another reason to choose exercise over the television!

Finally, additional research has shown that exercise can also help alleviate more specific negative symptoms, such as anger, confusion, fatigue and tension, with greater effects in people who are already classified as depressed.[23]

Study results like these are even more incredible when you consider that the worldwide market for antidepressants stands at about $20 billion. Not only is exercise cheaper, but it also doesn't have any other unpleasant side effects that medications can give you. This does not mean that antidepressants are not ever indicated, and they certainly serve a purpose in more severe forms of depression. But for more mild symptoms, we have to ask why society reaches for pills so easily when there is a proven therapy that is more fun, more self-satisfying and ultimately healthier? It's a culture I see on a daily basis in the medical world, among both physicians and patients. We as a society medicalize mild depression symptoms much too easily. There are natural fluctuations in everyone's lives and pills that can knock us out are not necessarily the right answer.

Improving your intelligence and brain health

It makes sense that an endorphin boost will also leave you able to think more clearly and enhance your mental performance. A survey of more than 250 students found that the grade point average (GPA) was 0.4 points higher on a 4.0 scale in those who exercised daily compared with those who didn't exercise.[24] Another review of more than 1 million men in Sweden found that cardiovascular fitness at age 18 predicted educational achievements later in life.[25]

This direct positive effect on the brain has also been found to apply to degenerative neurological conditions. A study that followed 300 older people for over a decade revealed that those who walked the most had an almost *50 percent reduced* risk of dementia signs such as memory loss.[26] The optimal amount of walking appeared to be between six and nine miles a week. The investigators also performed brain scans and, amazingly, found that the brains of those who walked the most were larger too. A similar effect was observed again in a group of 120 older volunteers who were asked to either walk around a track for 40 minutes a day, three days a week, or just do simple stretching exercises.[27] By the end of one year, MRI scans showed that the walking group had a 2 percent increase in hippocampus volume (a region of the brain involved in memory). On the contrary, the other group had a 1.4 percent *decrease* in volume, which is the same observed with normal aging. Therefore, it's no exaggeration to say that exercise really can help your brain to grow bigger.

Incorporating exercise into your life

These terrific health benefits of exercise are there for the taking. Even if you can't meet the minimum recommendations, something is always better than nothing. If you can do more than the minimum, that's a superb effort. The first step—if you don't already engage in regular physical activity—is to find something that you enjoy. There's so much to choose from. Are you a jogger, a swimmer, a tennis player? Do you like a variety of activities? Now work out if what you do is classed as moderate or vigorous activity. For instance, if you like to run, then this would typically be vigorous activity. If you have a mixture of a moderate activity like brisk walking combined with swimming, then that's fine too. Plan out your typical schedule and work out a good time to incorporate the activity into your week. Can you go to the gym before work, or are the evenings better for you? Make a plan and then try to hold yourself to it. If you want to jog several times a week, then make sure on most weeks you stick to it. If soccer club meets twice a week and you play for an hour each time, then stick to that. Either way, it should become part of your regular life schedule, much the same way that eating and sleeping are. There will always be excuses, like being busy with other commitments or having exams to study for. In fact, being busy with other things is even more of a reason to have a set exercise routine in order to reap the psychological benefits! When you make exercise part of your regular schedule, it will become like second nature. Try keeping count of whether you've had the minimum exercise time for the week. Once you get into it, you will likely go well over this time anyway as you begin to enjoy exercising more. Sports are especially good this way, because if you play a game of tennis or basketball for a couple of hours, that's already over a week of the recommended amount. And if you have health issues, like a bad knee, shoulder or back, then there are still other exercises you can do that can work around your problem. Swimming is a great exercise if you have a condition like osteoarthritis because your weight is supported by the water and the force you are putting through your joints is less than with running on the ground. Machines like ellipticals and cycling machines also put less strain on the joints.

Engaging in physical activity should never be viewed as a chore or a drag. If that's happening, then something is wrong, because it should be a part of your day that you relish and look forward to. One study from Sweden even looked into the importance of enjoyment in two exercise groups.[28] Using scientific algorithms, the researchers immediately found a strong association between enjoyment and exercise level. However, they also found associations between *changes* in enjoyment and *changes* in exercise level. It may sound like a no-brainer, but you have to enjoy it to be more likely to do it. So if you find jogging or cycling boring, then start to look for other forms of exercise that you are more fond of. You can also do other things to make exercise more fun. Try listening to your favorite music while you are running on the treadmill or cycling on the machine. This worked for me personally, as I found that using my iPod while running meant that I was happy doing it for much longer—because I was enjoying listening to my favorite tunes at the same time!

The process of getting exercise to be a regular part of your life may be a long one, but it's worth the time and effort. Want to exercise because you know it makes you feel good. Join a gym or a sports club; it's far better to spend the money here than on any other sedentary activity. Be aware when you haven't exercised for a while and feel the urge to get out there. It's a total win-win game.

HIGH PERCENTAGE ACTIVITY WELLNESS STEPS

- Keep in mind the weekly recommendations

    Distinguish between moderate and vigorous activity

- Join the gym

    Stick to a regular routine

- Take up a sport

    Find one you really enjoy

- Brisk walking is great

    You can do this at any time

- Exercise during your workday

    Take advantage of any small opportunities you can find

- Take the stairs

    Avoid elevators if you're only going up or down a flight or two

- Use exercise as a mood boost

    If you're feeling down, get those endorphins flowing

- Make sure exercise is always fun

    You can listen to music or join an exercise group

CHAPTER THREE

WEIGHT WELLNESS: SHEDDING THOSE POUNDS

Do you dread getting on the scales? You're not alone. According to figures from the CDC, more than two-thirds of all adults over the age of 20 are overweight or obese. This is more than double the rate of three decades ago. These dismal statistics are following similar trends across the world, as living standards increase and people eat more and more food. Current estimates put the number of obese people at 1 in 10 of the *world* population, which equates to 700 million people.[1] More worrisome, the problem is escalating in children too, with 20 percent of 6- to 11-year-olds and 10 percent of 2- to 5-year-olds being obese.[2] If this pattern continues, it is projected that a whopping 86 percent of us could be overweight or obese within twenty years![3]

Aside from the significant health and well-being drawbacks of these statistics, there is the additional drain on countries' finances. Studies have estimated that obesity costs the United States as much as $270 billion a year.[4] This comes in the form of increased healthcare costs and lost productivity. At the same time, many of us are painfully aware that we need to lose weight. A telephone survey of almost 185,000 people revealed that 46 percent of women and 33 percent of men reported current weight loss attempts.[5] The government is also now heeding the message, and is increasingly pushing initiatives that promote lifestyle changes. One example is with school meals, where there is tremendous room for improvement.

So far we have gone through the importance of healthy eating and getting enough exercise, both of which are obviously key factors in achieving a healthy weight. Many of the positive effects—such as lowered risk of heart disease and diabetes—that you have learned about in the previous chapters are directly linked to maintaining optimal body weight. One study of more than 7,000 middle-aged men who were followed for 20 years calculated that overweight people who lost weight could reduce their cardiovascular risk by up to *58 percent*.[6] In reality, getting to—and maintaining—an ideal weight is a big battle for most of us. There are very few people who are lucky enough to eat whatever they want and get away with no exercise, managing to have a great body shape and weight (and if there are, we all hate them anyway!). Like everything else in life, hard work and effort is the key 99 percent of the time.

I spend a lot of time hearing patients describe their ongoing struggles with weight. *But doctor, I eat really healthy food all the time and do loads of exercise, but still can't lose those excess pounds! I've tried everything and can't lose weight! Being overweight runs in my family!* You probably know people who have said similar things to you. The science tells us to be skeptical when we hear these stories. Sure, there are some medical conditions, like low thyroid function or other hormonal disorders, for example, that can make weight loss difficult, if not virtually impossible. If you believe you could be suffering from one of these, then get checked out by your doctor. For most people, however, this will not be the case. The majority of us are not hampered in reaching that optimal weight by a genuine medical problem. For those who blame being overweight on their family, it's certainly true that genetic predisposition to a certain body shape can make weight loss more difficult for some, but it's also just as likely that their situation is due to a poor lifestyle which their whole family is engaging in. Much larger influences come from our environment and habits, both of which are directly under our control.

Unfortunately, doctors are notoriously bad at addressing the issue of weight management with their patients. In spite of the epidemic-like figures, surveys have shown that more than 70 percent of overweight adults have never been advised to lose weight by their physicians or other healthcare practitioners.[7] Could you imagine the furor if other public health problems—like hypertension or diabetes—were being ignored like this? Ironically, it's been shown that people who do receive advice have almost *three times the odds* of actually trying to lose weight.[8] It appears that many physicians have simply given up trying. Maybe it's a bit of embarrassment too, because statistics show that doctors are often among the worst offenders, with close to 45 percent being overweight themselves.[9] It's always a bit difficult and uninspiring for anyone, not just a doctor, to give weight loss advice while their belly is hanging over their pants! As Laurence Fishburne said to Keanu Reeves in "The Matrix," *There's a difference between knowing the path and walking the path.*

The energy gap

When it comes to achieving a healthy weight, the simple and crucial concept to keep in mind is known as your *energy gap*.

(Energy input) minus (energy output)

If your input is consistently *more* than your output, you will always tend to put on weight. If the reverse is true, you will *lose* weight. It's that simple. For all the diet fads and exercising, for all those smaller portions, and all the times you pass on dessert, this is the very basic equation behind putting on or losing weight. When I encounter patients who are failing to lose the pounds despite claims of a healthy lifestyle, I remind them of their energy gap. This equation determines whether your body produces or burns off fat.

Since energy input is determined only by the food we eat, it is therefore the primary factor in determining our weight—more so than exercise in this respect. Prior surveys have, in fact, shown that many people who exercise regularly believe they have "earned" the right to eat almost whatever they like. Putting in all that effort to burn 400 hundred calories during that 30-minute run means nothing, in weight loss terms, if you go and eat a thousand-calorie dinner immediately afterwards. It may sound obvious, but this is where a lot of people who complain about their inability to lose weight fall behind. If your aim is to lose weight, your total input from food always has to be *less* than your output. If you want to avoid putting on weight, then input and output have to be consistently equal.

Also bear in mind that your ability to lose weight depends partly on your gender and age. Women may think this horribly unfair, but men are able to lose more weight than women of a similar size because they have more lean body mass and lower body fat, which results in higher energy expenditure. As we age, our metabolic rate also declines by approximately 2 percent every decade, which tends to make weight loss even harder. In these respects, older women have the most raw deal!

Body mass index and waist-to-hip ratio

You've probably already heard the term *body mass index* to describe how healthy someone's weight is. This is a mathematical calculation that you can easily figure out on yourself. In scientific terms, it is your weight in kilograms divided by your height in meters squared. Before you rush for your calculator, there are numerous websites that can calculate this for you in a few seconds. This is what the numbers mean:

Underweight = <18.5
Normal weight = 18.5–24.9
Overweight = 25–29.9
Obesity = BMI of 30 or greater

A second measure to know is your *waist-to-hip ratio*. Using a measuring tape, measure the circumference of your hips at the widest part and then measure your waist circumference at or just above the belly button. To calculate the ratio, divide your waist measurement by your hip measurement. A healthy waist-to-hip ratio for women is 0.8 or lower. A healthy ratio for men is 1.0 or lower. In other words, your waist should be *less* than your hips. Ratios above 0.8 for women and 1.0 for men are indicative of obesity. The higher the ratio, the bigger your belly. Medical research indicates that this ratio can actually be more important to your health than your total weight or body mass index, both of which can be influenced by other factors such as bone density. In layman's terms, people who gain weight mostly on their hips and buttocks are termed "pear-shaped," while people who tend to gain weight on their abdomen are called "apple-shaped." One team from Canada analyzed data from close to 10,000 adults and found that waist circumference was the single biggest indicator of heart disease risk.[10] Other research from the University of Texas followed over 700 people for more than seven years.[11] During this time, more than 100 new cases of diabetes were diagnosed. The researchers calculated that having a larger waist circumference was the biggest predictor of developing diabetes, the risk being an astonishing *11 times greater* for those with the largest waist circumference compared to those with the lowest. So it's not all about your absolute weight. Body fat distribution and waist-to-hip ratio are critical as well.

On a superficial note, while we are on the subject, there have been a number of studies performed on female attractiveness in terms of body shape. Scientists have consistently found that a waist-to-hip ratio of 0.7 is always seen as the most attractive across different cultures and countries![12]

Tipping the energy gap in your favor

The first step in losing weight is to control your calorie intake. As you read in Chapter One, the amount we take in on a routine basis has grown significantly over the years. I'm always struck when I visit other countries by how much smaller their portions are. Our medium size is another country's large size, and most other countries don't even have a "super size." You cannot be habitually eating high-calorie meals if you want to lose weight. There are literally hundreds of recommended diets, from low-carbohydrate to almost zero-fat, which claim to be the solution to your weight-loss woes. Some declare that you will not even notice a difference in your regular routine. Others insist that you can even feel more full while actually losing weight. All of them, however, have one thing in common. They are all about reducing caloric intake and tipping the energy balance in your favor. We've already talked about nutritious eating, and generally, if you are eating a healthy, balanced diet, you will be well placed to lose weight with a little bit of extra effort.

The traditional view has always just been to stick to a low-fat diet. This is because in simple terms, fat contains the most calories. One gram of fat contains 9 calories, compared to one gram of carbohydrate or protein, which both contain 4 calories each. In the last couple of decades especially, many new diets have emerged that suggest other alternatives. Rather than just believe all of the hype, let's look at some of the evidence and review the science.

The evidence for different diets

Low-carbohydrate diets became popular with the advent of the well-known Atkins Diet. Stories of dramatic weight loss have been well-portrayed in the media. But how do low-carb diets stack up against low-fat diets? Certainly in the short term, low-carbohydrate, high-protein diets can be successful in producing weight loss for several months. Over the longer term though, the evidence is more debatable. A team from Stanford University conducted a study that compared four popular low-calorie diets that varied according to carbohydrate and fat content.[13] More than 300 overweight and obese women were randomly assigned to follow one of the diets. The results showed that after one year, the women in the lowest carbohydrate group had lost the most weight, on average 4.7 kilograms (10.4 pounds). This was more than *50 percent greater* than the high-carbohydrate, low-fat diet. The women also exhibited other improved parameters such as better HDL "good" cholesterol and blood pressure.

In another experiment, researchers from Temple University again took 300 obese volunteers and placed them on either a low-carbohydrate or low-fat diet (less than 30 percent energy from fat).[14] Both groups also received a lifestyle modification program. After two years, there were *no* significant differences in weight loss in either group. Both had lost an impressive average of 11 kilograms (24.3 pounds) at one year, and 7 kilograms (15.4 pounds) at two years. However, like the Stanford study, the low-carbohydrate group was found to have improvements in their HDL cholesterol of almost 25 percent.

A more extensive analysis was published in the *New England Journal of Medicine*, comparing four different weight-loss diets in 800 adults.[15] This time, it was found that after six months people on each diet had lost an average of 6 kilograms (13.2 pounds), although in general they began to regain the weight after one year. By two years, weight loss was similar in the high- and low-fat, high- and low-protein, and most importantly the high- and low-carbohydrate diets. Overall, among those who completed the trial, the average weight loss was 4 kilograms (8.8 pounds). The study concluded that all the diets could result in significant weight loss no matter which macronutrients were consumed. The most important thing was to *reduce* your calories.

So as you can see, both low-carbohydrate and low-fat diets can help you shed the pounds, as long as total calorie intake is reduced. One reason why low-carbohydrate diets work is that many of these involve higher protein intake, which has been found to reduce hunger and significantly reduce food intake, especially during the short-term.[16] When carbohydrate intakes are very low (less than 20 grams per day), as is the case with the Atkins' Diet, the body's glycogen stores are mobilized due to reduced glucose availability. Fat breakdown occurs, which causes accumulation of molecules called ketone bodies, leading to what's known as a *ketogenic state*. Fluid loss also takes place, which aids the weight loss. This is not without potential side effects, and these diets can been associated with unpleasant symptoms such as headaches and cramps. Although the changes in the "good" HDL cholesterol appear to favor low-carbohydrate diets, these have to be taken in context with the fact that low-fat diets are much more likely to produce improved LDL "bad" cholesterol levels.

The best advice is somewhere in the middle of the road. If you want to lose weight, cut back sensibly on both bad fats and bad carbohydrates. If you decide that a more restrictive diet is what you need, be advised that this may not be sustainable for long periods of time. Whichever one you choose, remember that the underlying principles are based on biology and physiology, and are simply working at tipping the energy balance equation negatively. Most importantly, stick to the diet for long enough to notice the effects. A week-long crash diet is nonsensical. Like evidence-based eating in general, if you make the changes part of your regular routine, they will be more likely to work and reap you long-term rewards.

Feeling full and drinking water

One of the reasons why dieting can seem painful is that we are often left not feeling full. A feeling of satiety is a basic need for all of us. Physiologically, it takes about 20 minutes for our stomachs to get there, and you can actually take advantage of this biological fact in your dieting strategy. The most basic method is by ensuring that you don't eat too fast. The slower you can eat during a meal, the better. In a way, it's playing a trick on your stomach receptors. Eating a healthy starter about 20 to 30 minutes before a meal can serve the same purpose too. Something like an apple—which is high in fiber and low in calories—can contribute to earlier fullness. A team from Virginia Tech University conducted an experiment that looked into whether an even simpler method, drinking pure water, could also work.[17] The researchers divided almost 50 volunteer dieters into two groups. The first group adhered to a simple low-calorie diet; the second group followed the same diet, but drank two glasses of water, approximately half a liter (17 ounces), before each meal. After just 12 weeks, this latter group showed an incredible 44 *percent greater* decline in weight, which equated to 2 kilograms (4.4 pounds) more than the other group, mainly because they ate much less afterwards. Therefore, consuming approximately two cups of water prior to meals had a profound weight-loss effect. Water also has the additional benefit of having absolutely *no* calories. Be careful though—if you use this technique—not to over-hydrate yourself, which can be dangerous. One to two glasses should be just fine.

A further hidden advantage of drinking water is that every time you drink it, you are avoiding taking in something else that is potentially bad for you. Using more data from the Stanford weight loss study we discussed before, it was found that replacing sweetened beverages with water was associated with significant loss of body weight and fat, *independent* of other variables such as diet type and physical activity.[18] The authors calculated that increasing water intake to more than one liter a day was associated with significant weight loss over 12 months, equivalent to an annual energy expenditure of 17,400 calories. A huge amount of hidden calories are taken in every day through what we drink—up to 10 percent of total energy intake through sweetened drinks. Drinking pure water instead is an easy way to eliminate some of these calories and tip the energy balance further in your favor. If you find water boring, add a slice of lemon or lime or a few drops of lemon juice and pour over ice—that's one of my personal favorites!

Awareness

We said in the first chapter that *awareness* is key. If you don't know what you are taking in, then obviously you won't be in any position to control it. Even something as simple as reading food labels can have a dramatic effect on whether or not you are likely to succeed in losing weight. One study from the University of Washington asked more than 3,700 dieters whether they read food labels, and found that those who did so had a much better chance of weight loss.[19] Curiously, this effect applied especially to women. The researchers also found that label readers who did not exercise had a greater chance of losing weight compared with people who exercised but did not read labels.

The Nutrition Labeling and Education Act of 1994 requires all food manufacturers to present standardized nutrition facts on the package, so this is an easy enough thing for us to do in the supermarket. Most labels present both the total amount, and to be more convenient, the *amount per serving*. Read them next time you're buying groceries. Take care that the amount per serving is actually what you are going to be eating, because sometimes the bar is placed very low to make the product sound better. For instance, a processed food item that is really only enough for one person in one sitting may be displayed on the label as being two or three "servings." You may think a serving of, let's say, cookies is the whole package (especially with these mini-bags that have become so popular), when in reality, the serving is much less than you might think. That's why it pays to read the labels!

Some restaurants are following suit too. I've been to several eating establishments in bigger cities that have started displaying calorie counts on the menu. It would be a revolution if this were made compulsory, as most people would instantly think twice before ordering. Restaurants are unlikely though to be such big fans of this practice, for obvious reasons. Most of their popular money-making dishes might overnight become less popular if calorie counts were displayed openly. After all, who would really be keen on eating that 600- calorie dessert? But on the other side of the coin, it could also be a great opportunity for restaurants to develop and promote healthier options. Perhaps it'll happen one day.

Visualization

Being able to actually see your progress can either be very encouraging or a push to try even harder. Keeping a dietary record is another simple method that can greatly enhance your chances of success. A survey conducted by the University of Oregon of almost 1,700 overweight and obese adult dieters showed that people who kept daily food records lost almost *twice as much* weight as those who didn't.[20] You don't need to be obsessive about recording every single crumb you consume, but keeping a good account in a food diary of what you are eating will help you to assess exactly how much you are taking in and where you might be going wrong. The same principle applies to keeping a visual weight record. If you see that the trend is upwards, it can motivate you to try harder. If the trend is downwards, it encourages you to keep going. Write down your weight every week or two in a logbook. Alternatively, draw a chart on a whiteboard, and place it somewhere in your house that you can see it (obviously away from where every nosey guest might also see it!). If you can, also note down your body mass index and body fat percentage. The more you keep track, the better. Don't underestimate the motivation you can get from a simple visual cue of your progress. Along the same lines, other studies have shown that keeping big mirrors around your house, especially in the kitchen, can also help you monitor yourself more effectively and adopt better eating habits.[21]

And sticking with this visualization theme, a fascinating experiment showed that even just *imagining* eating high-calorie foods could be enough to stop you indulging in them. Researchers at Carnegie Mellon University asked a group of volunteers to imagine eating 30 M&Ms, after which they were actually instructed to eat some from a bowl.[22] When compared to a control group that didn't imagine eating any, these people were consistently found to eat fewer M&Ms! The investigators concluded that a simple mental representation may reduce our subsequent desire to eat bad foods, contradicting the traditionally held view that thinking about things makes us crave them more.

Reducing access

The concept of actually *reducing* access sounds foreign because in most areas of life we are concerned with always *increasing* access. But with bad foods, this is usually a good move. The more that a potentially tasty but high-calorie meal or snack is in front of you, the more tempted you will be to grab it. As humans we are prone to eating what's easily accessible whenever we are hungry. If you don't buy high-calorie items in the first place, then you won't be able to eat them when you get hungry. It is a simple technique that can be very effective. Even away from home, the same is true whether you are out and about, or at work. I know I always get hungry around mid-morning and mid-afternoon. I take in a banana and an apple every day to keep on my desk. When I get a bit hungry, I just grab these easily accessible options. They are not in my bag or in my office drawer. I have placed them strategically right there on my table, with no other food options immediately around me. This also ensures that I am eating healthy fruits every day instead of chocolate bars or potato chips. There was a news report when the Obama Administration took over the White House that they were trying to get people to eat healthier during the day by replacing bowls of candy with apples instead. The hope was that the busy staff who got hungry would grab apples instead of a handful of candies. That's a great idea.

Researchers from the University of Michigan highlighted how our environments can contribute to weight gain by conducting a study on college freshmen.[23] They specifically wanted to look at what effect dormitory eating arrangements would have on weight gain during that first year away from home. Their findings were sobering, if a little unsurprising. Students randomly assigned to residence halls with on-site dining facilities were clearly found to gain much more weight during their freshman year than those who lived in halls with no dining facilities. Females in these dorms were almost 1 kilogram (2.2 pounds) heavier by the end of the year. Males in these dorms consumed significantly more meals and more snacks. The researchers also found that females who lived closer to the campus gym automatically exercised more than those living farther away. This study was interesting because it was a natural experiment in otherwise healthy young people. It highlights two important points that apply across all ages, based on the principle of "access is key." First, having regular large meals at your disposal will mean that you will usually tend to eat them. Second, with any healthy behavior such as exercise, the easier it is for you to do, the more you will be inclined to do so. The bigger the barrier between yourself and the behavior, the easier it is to avoid.

We've all likely experienced this effect in our own lives. During my typical workday, I rarely eat three full meals. But when I was a medical student on rotations, we frequently used to get meal tokens to use at least three times a day in the hospital cafeteria. Now anyone who has ever been a student knows that a free token for anything is like manna from heaven. So what did we all do without fail three times a day? Of course we all sat together to dine and enjoy our free meals! Whether it's at an all-you-can-eat buffet at the local restaurant or on-board a cruise ship with 24/7 dining options, this is usually the case. If we have access to a large meal, we will almost always tend to overindulge when it is right in front of us.

How can you apply these findings to yourself? Fundamentally, as we've already said, not buying bad foods such as high calorie snacks in the first place is a great start. Simple rule—if it's not in your kitchen, you can't eat it. Never go to the grocery store hungry, because the chances of you putting those naughty snacks in your cart will be dramatically increased as the caveman in you will be leading you down the wrong aisles. When trying to lose weight, avoid buffet meals and limit yourself to restaurants only as a treat. At work, can you avoid going near the cafeteria or candy machine at the wrong times? It may be difficult to do, but the harder it is for you to get to, the less likely you are to eat there. Take some healthy fruits to work and leave them on your desk or in your locker. If you are studying or reading, can you do it as far away as possible from any tempting snacks? Anything that increases the barrier and reduces access will help you in your efforts to lose weight.

Avoiding the weekend blues

There are always times when we are more prone to letting ourselves go and having a bit of a splurge. That's not to suggest that if you are at a special occasion, you shouldn't eat well, but there are more frequent setbacks that people may be suffering in their weight-loss strategy. One such common scenario is for people to indulge themselves over the weekends, so much so that their hard work during the week is negated. Having been good all week, we become less disciplined on weekends. This is a disaster if you are trying to lose weight, because if you think about it, the weekend is almost *one-third* of the entire week! A study from Washington University took almost 50 adults and weighed them daily before, and during, a weight-loss trial.[24] The investigators found that prior to the study, participants on average lost weight during weekdays, but then consistently gained weight on the weekends. When they went further and analyzed dietary patterns and behaviors, they found that weekend weight gain was directly attributable to higher dietary intake (and also lower physical activity). And even when the participants were dieting, they still tended to stop losing weight over the weekends and put on the pounds instead.

Most of us work hard during the week and find it easier to keep relatively good habits. As soon as we get time off, things slip. Be careful that all your hard work is not undone over the weekend. We can ensure this by sticking as much as possible to our regular daily routine in terms of eating and physical exercise—yes, even on Saturdays and Sundays. You can still get up early (if you haven't been partying the night before) and replace your work routine with other chores. Get out of the house at a good time, get outdoors, visit friends...anything so you don't become sedentary and start munching on extra food at home. Try your best to maintain the same eating pattern that you had during the week. If you know you are going out for a big dinner, then have a light lunch or do extra exercise to maintain the energy balance situation.

Previous surveys have shown that holiday seasons are other potential pitfalls for dieters. But these times are relatively short-lived and infrequent, and it would not be very much fun to be too strict during these occasions. But, when we are dealing with weekends, it's a problem to drop the ball for that long if weight loss is the aim.

Cutting back on television time

In the last chapter, we touched upon the fact that we spend too much time watching television. On the bright side, TV programs are great sources of information and entertainment that have greatly enriched our lives. Nonetheless, they do have one major drawback that is impossible to rectify. The process of viewing a television screen is an entirely *sedentary* activity. To make things twice as bad, we also tend to eat junk food and snack as we are sitting in front of the box. In a study from Strasbourg, France, researchers looked at the association between adolescents having a television in their bedroom and their lifestyle habits.[25] Almost 380 twelve-year-old children were studied for three years, with the presence or absence of a television set in the bedroom, and details on other leisure activities, assessed by questionnaire. Each child underwent an annual physical assessment. The results should make any parent sit up and take notice. First, both boys and girls who had a TV in their room reported reading much less. Second, there was a clear and direct relationship between having a TV and obesity levels, and this was especially significant in boys. Interestingly, this was not solely associated with less physical activity, meaning that other issues such as snacking were also a likely issue. Today, it is estimated that two-thirds of adolescents have a television in their bedrooms. Maybe it's time to take these away.

How to become the biggest loser

Weight is one situation where boasting that you are the biggest loser can be a good thing! Just from looking around we know that some people are much better at achieving it than others. In fact, one of the biggest problems with losing weight is failure to maintain it in the long-term. We put all that effort into shedding those pounds, and then so many people just put it right back on again. What are the key factors that determine success versus failure? Researchers from Pittsburgh attempted to answer this question by investigating a group of people who had already been successful in their weight-loss endeavors.[26] More than 700 volunteers were studied who had lost at least 13.6 kilograms (30 pounds) and had maintained this weight loss for at least one year. Standardized questionnaires documented weight, dietary habits, activity and psychological characteristics over the course of the year. By this time, a disappointing 35 percent had regained an average of 7 kilograms. However, almost 60 percent had been successful in maintaining their weight loss. The rest had actually managed to lose even more weight. When the researchers took a closer look at those who were successful versus those who weren't, they found the risk factors for weight regain included people who initially had more rapid and larger weight losses before the study, higher levels of dietary disinhibition (less restraint), a tendency to binge eat and depression. Maintainers tended to be much more disciplined and stick to constant behaviors. The weight gainers also had a significant decline in self-monitoring habits and less energy expenditure through physical activity. This confirms what should be obvious by now. Failure to maintain the right behaviors quickly reverses all that great work. As soon as you let go and get back to those bad old habits, you've had it. This was the same discovery that another multicenter team made when they asked similar questions to a group of almost 475 overweight or obese people.[27] Their results showed that the biggest factors in successful weight loss were dietary restraint and higher total physical activity. When they analyzed the environmental factors that contributed to failure, there were associations with having high-fat foods at home, lack of access to exercise equipment and—yes, number of televisions at home!

Finally, to nail home the point in more detail, the CDC used data from mail surveys to determine the lifestyle patterns in almost 2,000 adults who had attempted to lose weight.[28] Their answers revealed that successful people were more likely to plan their meals, track their own calories, monitor fat intake, measure their food on a plate, find cooking and baking fun (probably because that meant they would eat more at home), and weigh themselves daily—almost *10 percent more likely* in all these categories. The investigators also found that people who ate out often or found healthy foods too expensive were *48 to 64 percent less successful*, and that those who reported no time or felt too tired to exercise were *48 to 76 percent less successful*. Intriguingly too, the best weight losers were actually *less* likely to use over-the-counter diet products, proving that looking for "quick diet fixes" is not the answer if you don't maintain all the other right behaviors.

Motivating yourself

The missing link so far, arguably the most important factor, is the simple concept of *motivation*. You have to be driven to lose weight. You really, *really* have to want to do it. Without getting ahead of myself, because we'll talk a bit more about life motivation in general in a future chapter, it's clearly the crucial ingredient. A joint study by the Universities of Kentucky and North Carolina looked at the two types of motivation involved in weight loss, known as *autonomous* and *controlled*.[29] Psychological questionnaires were administered to almost 70 volunteers during a four-month weight loss trial. People who were motivated by factors such as feeling that "performance is the best way to help themselves" and wanting to lose weight for personal reasons, were exhibiting something known as *autonomous motivation*. People who were motivated only by external controls such as pressure from others were exhibiting *controlled motivation*. The participants also had to regularly record their diet, exercise and body weight. Overall, more than 50 percent of participants lost at least 5 percent of their initial body weight after 16 weeks—an impressive result. When the researchers looked at the data further, they found that most of the participants had a significant increase in both autonomous and controlled motivation during the first four weeks of the study. There was, however, a direct relationship between weight loss at four weeks and higher autonomic motivation, when compared to people with higher levels of controlled motivation. People who went on to achieve at least a 5 percent weight loss were more likely to have sustained autonomous motivation between 4 and 16 weeks. In contrast, the people who were less successful experienced a significant decrease in both forms of motivation. Overall, autonomous motivation after four weeks was found to be a significant predictor of increased self-monitoring and weight loss. This makes sense too. Wanting to do something for yourself always wins.

So how can you increase your own internal autonomic motivation? Well, if learning about the terrific health benefits of weight loss and having a better body shape isn't enough for you, then maybe nothing will be!

Your weight loss strategy

You need to have firm determination if you want to reach and maintain your weight goal. Work out your own personal dieting strategy based on nutrition content and other lifestyle techniques. Like any other big project, whether it's buying a home or planning an event, it requires organization, the right oversight and persistence. One survey of more than 1,800 obese adults enrolled in a weight-loss trial showed that those people who had a specific strategy, such as reducing calories, decreasing fat intake or increasing exercise, were much more likely to achieve weight loss two years later.[30] Conversely, those who did not engage in a strategy tended to gain weight instead.

Keep telling yourself that you can and will get to that desired weight. Visualize yourself fitting into those clothes you've always wanted to, having a flatter belly and receiving compliments on how much weight you've lost. If you are faced with a tempting choice that is taking you away from your strategy, remember the old saying, *a minute on the lips, a lifetime on the hips!* Supermodel Kate Moss was widely criticized not long ago for making the statement, "Nothing tastes as good as skinny feels." The worry from the media was that this would encourage young women to become anorexic, which is a devastating medical condition. However, if we don't take the extreme example, what she said has a ring of truth to it. Being an overweight couch potato is also potentially devastating too. Getting in better shape brings all sorts of health benefits, plus the internal satisfaction that you will feel. If you already have an ideal weight and are happy with it, then congratulations, this chapter wasn't so much for you. But the statistics suggest that you are becoming the minority. It's not all about being thin either, but more about just being a healthy weight.

A common misconception is that people need to go hungry in order to lose weight. If you are following a diet like that to get to where you want, then it's a recipe for just losing it and then putting it back on again, which we've seen is an all too common occurrence. You don't need to go hungry at all. You can even *add* things to your diet and still lose weight as long as you cut out the bad stuff. Avoid at all costs one of those notorious crash diets. When you starve yourself or skip meals, your body goes into survival mode and actually fights to preserve energy, slowing down your metabolic rate. This can conversely even lead to you *putting on* weight. One example is skipping breakfast, which research shows just leads to later hunger, making it more difficult to lose weight.[31] Far better to eat regularly, but be more careful about what you are eating. It's even okay to eat four or five smaller meals a day if that works for you, rather than eating fewer but larger meals. This can actually help boost your metabolism, producing better weight loss. Furthermore, always eat your dinner at least three hours before sleeping, which will give your meals more time to digest while your metabolism is high.

Having a regular routine is also great for weight management. If you have spare time to sit around, you often tend to eat. You also have more time to think about eating. Have you ever been so busy and caught up that you realized it was a couple of hours after your normal eating time? Your body will, of course, tell you when it's time to eat, but it just goes to show how we often don't even need to eat. Eat only when you're hungry.

Set yourself small targets for weight loss. It's completely unrealistic and usually futile to say that you are going to lose 20 pounds in just a few weeks. Instead, aim for a pound every couple of weeks, which is much more achievable. When I talk to patients, they will usually be thinking in terms of these large increments. Ironically, doctors make the same mistake too. It should not be about saying, "Sir, you need to lose 20 pounds." That's only the final target. Set small goals, where you can notice the improvements and feel good about achieving them. You may think that losing a pound at a time is hardly noticeable, but if you consistently go about it, and notice a downward trend over time (on your weight loss whiteboard), you will soon feel encouraged. It will be rewarding to step on those scales and see the fruits of your hard work. Imagine that instead of dreading stepping on the scales every week, you looked *forward* to it and were expecting good results. Keep viewing your weight loss as a journey and not just a temporary phase.

If you find it difficult to do on your own, make a pact with a friend or family member in the same situation as you. Join a weight-loss group. Millions have had success this way. If we are surrounded by the right role models, then we are more likely to go the same way too. It's not easy to lose weight, but then nothing that's desirable ever is. Even if there were a pill that could get people to their ideal weight in an instant, that wouldn't necessarily be a good thing. If such a medication existed, it would enable people to carry on eating badly and remaining sedentary. Being overweight is the warning from your body that things need to change.

HIGH PERCENTAGE WEIGHT WELLNESS STEPS

- Get used to thinking in terms of your daily energy gap

    Energy input should not be more than output

- Regularly measure your weight

    Buy a scale that also measures body mass index (BMI) and body fat percentage

- Keep track of your waist-to-hip ratio

    You can easily measure this on yourself

- Both low-fat and low-carbohydrate diets can work

    Choose whichever one works for you

- Limit portions but avoid going hungry for long

    Smaller but more frequent meals are okay

- Feel full earlier

    Eat more slowly, have a high-fiber appetizer, and drink plenty of water

- Read food labels and keep a dietary record

    Monitoring intake is crucial

- Keep a visual record of your weight

    Buy a diary or whiteboard to chart your progress

- Restrict your access to high-calorie foods

    Don't buy them in the first place!

- Maintain your healthy ways on weekends

    Avoid losing all your hard work on Saturdays and Sundays

- Limit your daily television viewing

    This is an entirely sedentary activity

- Choose to lose weight for yourself

    Be internally motivated to do it

- Have a definite strategy

    Stick to it and maintain those disciplined behaviors

CHAPTER FOUR

ENERGY WELLNESS: MAINTAINING THE BOOST

Every day millions of people complain of constantly feeling tired, with some estimates suggesting that about 25 percent of us suffer persistently low energy levels.[1] Many more people report fatigue levels that are seriously impairing their ability to perform daily tasks. As a consequence it is one of the most common reasons for physician visits, accounting for as many as 10 million a year.[2] This symptom has therefore become a major public health problem.

There are a number of medical problems that can cause us to feel tired, ranging from relatively minor to much more serious. If you find yourself feeling more lethargic than usual, always get checked out by your doctor first. Frequently though, when people report chronic lethargy, all of the blood tests and other imaging tests will return negative. It's then that we have to take an in-depth look at any lifestyle habits which may be contributing to the symptoms.

We all have natural energy highs and lows during the day. They fluctuate naturally along with our daily experiences and moods. Feeling energetic and full of vitality is impossible all the time. The word *vitality* is actually even more encompassing than energy, because it includes that sense of enthusiasm and aliveness too. There will always be intervals when you feel tired, and other times when you feel like you can take on the whole world. You may know some (usually a bit annoying!) people who are always jumping around throughout the day—however, this is not entirely natural either. But when your energy lows are making it difficult for you to function at the level you want, then you have a problem. If you find yourself feeling tired and jaded on most days, there may be a few simple things you can do to pick yourself back up.

Eating the low-glycemic way

To recap from the first chapter, the *glycemic index* refers to the change in blood glucose levels produced by what you eat. You've probably already noticed yourself feeling lethargic after eating certain meals, but exactly what you eat is the determining factor in whether or not it is likely to make you feel tired. Foods that cause a rapid spike in blood sugar are much worse than foods which result in a more steady rise. That's yet another reason to prefer low-glycemic foods. A combined British and Australian team designed a study that mimics many of the breakfast choices we face, and their subsequent effects on our energy levels throughout the morning.[3] Fourteen volunteer students were given four different breakfasts on separate mornings, each containing the same number of calories. Two of the breakfasts were high in carbohydrates and low in fat. One of these contained low-glycemic index carbohydrates and high-fiber (all-bran) and the other, high-glycemic index carbohydrates and lower fiber (cornflakes). The other two breakfasts were high in fat and low in fiber (croissants with spread, and eggs with bacon). For the rest of the day, each participant completed questionnaires and filled out diaries that assessed appetite and alertness ratings at regular intervals, and also recorded all fluid and food intake. When the results were analyzed, the researchers found some stark differences in how the breakfasts made people feel. The high-fiber, all-bran meal produced the highest post-breakfast alertness ratings, about *70 percent more* than the high-fat breakfasts. This increased alertness persisted at all times up to lunch. In contrast, the high-glycemic index cornflakes breakfast resulted in declining alertness ratings. The all-bran breakfast also produced more subjective feelings of fullness, and the least subsequent food intake up until lunch. On average, the participants waited almost *50 percent longer* before eating again after all-bran compared to when eating eggs and bacon. The exact order of the alertness ratings were: all-bran (most alert), followed by cornflakes, eggs and bacon, and croissants (least alert). The message from this study was clear. To stay most alert during the morning, eat a low-glycemic index, fiber-rich breakfast—which we already know is the most healthy as well. It's also much better for weight loss as it's more filling and leaves our hunger more satisfied.

The same principle applies just as equally when choosing what to eat for lunch, which is especially important if you are working or attending school. In fact, the phenomenon known as *post-lunch lethargy* or the *mid-afternoon slump* is attracting the attention of the business community, because it is estimated to cost companies billions of dollars a year. If you find yourself falling asleep in the middle of the afternoon, it may be your lunch and not just your dull desk job! In one experiment, researchers took 12 adults and fed them three different lunches.[4] After eating, they all underwent computer reaction and concentration testing. The results showed that a lunch higher in protein resulted in better performance compared to a high-carbohydrate lunch.

And how about those brief moments during the day when you feel a bit sluggish? Lots of people look for a quick sugar fix when this happens. Be careful if this is your strategy, because something like a chocolate bar will have the same temporary effect in causing rapid blood sugar fluctuations—a quick rise followed by a rapid crash. The same goes for sugar loaded drinks, which have been found to *not* counteract sleepiness for very long, and ultimately lead to slower reaction times and poorer concentration.[5]

So if you want your diet to be compatible with maintaining high energy levels and performance during the day, eat only low-glycemic index foods, and avoid large quantities of carbohydrates. Try this experiment on yourself for two consecutive days. One day, eat a high-glycemic index breakfast or lunch and the next day go low-glycemic. Don't consume any high-sugar snacks or beverages during your workday. The science suggests you should notice a difference.

The great outdoors

Being outside in the fresh air and a natural environment can really help us rejuvenate. This is more than just an old wives' tale. In fact, research shows that even just *imagining* being outdoors or surrounding yourself with natural pictures can have a dramatic effect on your energy levels! An international team of researchers conducted a large experiment that looked into how nature, both perceived and experienced, really affects us.[6] First, they asked a group of more than 170 undergraduate students to imagine themselves in certain situations, including being outdoors, and then rate their energy, vitality and alertness using a scientific scale. The results showed conclusively that the students reported significantly *higher* levels of vitality when imagining themselves being outside. In total contrast, students who had to imagine themselves being alone and inactive had much *lower* levels of vitality. And this was just using their imagination. The researchers then showed a group of almost 100 students images of either nature, such as a lake, or manmade images like a building or street, for two minutes. Again, the students who were shown the nature pictures reported an *increase* in vitality, while those who viewed the building slides actually had a *decrease* in vitality. To further substantiate the findings and make things more practical, groups were then asked to walk either inside or outside for 15 minutes. The outdoor group walked along a tree-lined footpath next to a river. When the researchers looked at the results of the same energy and vitality scale, they found that indoor walking had no effect on vitality, whereas outdoor walking produced another significant *increase* in vitality. Finally, to gain even more insight, another group of almost 140 students were asked to keep diaries of their activities for two weeks, and would randomly receive a pager call during the day to confirm what they were doing (it's surprising how much inconvenience some students will go through to earn some extra cash in a research study!). Once more, it was found that the participants consistently felt more energized when outdoors, with an especially greater sense of vitality on days when they spent at least 20 minutes outdoors. But that was not all. Further detailed analyses revealed that there was a difference between being outdoors and being in nature. Namely, the presence of nature appeared to have an *independent* energizing effect above that of being outdoors. Taking an outdoor mountain walk was better than taking an outdoor walk along a busy street.

Not surprisingly, the type of weather can also have a large effect on us. It makes a big difference whether we are outdoors in the sun or outdoors in the clouds and rain. In a study conducted in Michigan, participants were randomly assigned to either being outside on warm and sunny spring days, outside on unpleasant days, or indoors.[7] Using standardized testing, the people who were outside on warm and clearer days reported better mood and memory. To experience the maximum benefit, it appears we need at least 30 minutes outside in this type of weather. Does this mean that those of us who live in New England should be packing our bags and moving South? It may not be ideal for a lot of us (although judging by the people I've met, many who live up here would be lying if they said the thought hadn't crossed their minds before), but some sunny and warm weather as often as you are able to get it is a great idea.

And even when we do find ourselves stuck indoors, we can add some nature to our surroundings. As well as hanging pictures depicting nature, just surrounding ourselves with other natural items can reap us more dividends. Research shows that flowers, for instance, can work to give us a boost. In an interesting experiment, more than 50 adults were investigated to find out the potential effect on the psyche of having flowers in the home.[8] The volunteers were divided into two groups, one receiving flowers at home in a room they frequented often, and the second receiving another home décor item. Over the course of a week, as well as having other beneficial effects on mood, it was found that those with flowers at home also experienced a boost of energy and enthusiasm that managed to carry over to their work environment. One good thing about our inner caveman is this attraction to natural things, as there's something in our innate biology that will always like being around nature.

How can you apply all of these findings to your own life to take advantage of these energizing properties of nature? For a start, you can try to get outdoors as much as possible. Even during your workday, is there any way you can just sneak outside for a quick walk in the fresh air? Even if you're downtown with no natural surroundings, being outdoors will still do you good. If you can go somewhere more natural—near a lake perhaps, or a forest path, or a mountainside, that's even better. If it's not possible during the day, aim for a regular amount of nature on evenings and weekends. Think of it as a dose of pleasant medication that will give you a boost. Make the interior of your house or office more natural too. Hang pictures of nature and add some plants. By making your office or your homework space somewhere that you find really soothing, you will enjoy being there more, and likely be more productive too. When you are doing other work that needs you to be at your peak, such as studying for an exam or doing a project on your laptop, work outside if it's a nice day. I knew a lot of university friends who would sit outside in the summer and study. I'm ashamed to say that in my ignorance, I never used to, but I totally would now.

Having said all of this, when you do get outside, statistics show that you may be in the minority, because it's estimated that people in the Western world spend more than 90 percent of their time indoors. That's a great shame, and something you can help change right now.

Quick thinking to shift your brain into gear

Similar to revving the accelerator to get your car engine working, the same principle applies to your brain. We all occasionally get that mind-block where we feel devoid of energy and ideas. Our mind appears to have ground to a halt and is moving much more slowly than usual. Ironically, scientists have been gaining insight into a technique that may help us increase our own mind energy levels by looking into what the problem is in those who have abnormally high, uncontrollable energy levels, a condition known as *manic disorder*. People who suffer from this condition have racing thoughts and elevated mood associated with exhilaration and high energy levels. The question that some scientists have been posing turns this issue around 360 degrees. Can fast thinking in normal people bring about higher energy levels? In a joint study from Harvard and Princeton Universities, almost 150 students sat at a computer and were told to read a series of statements that appeared one word at a time on the screen.[9] Some of the statements contained positive undertones, and others were more negative. Some of the statements were read fast and others more slowly. After reading the statements, each student completed a detailed psychological evaluation. The results revealed that the fast-thinking group consistently experienced higher energy levels, positive mood, feelings of power, creativity and inspiration. Researchers found this effect regardless of whether the statements were positive or negative, and that it was fast thinking alone that produced the results. In other words, accelerated thought speed alone helped boost feelings of positive energy. The experiment also revealed that the participants had to be aware of their own thought speed in order to experience this effect. It has to be something you know you are doing, unlike those with manic disorder who don't have insight into their condition.

Other research has backed up these findings, showing that people who participate in activities that induce fast thinking—such as brainstorming for ideas, playing word games, or reading aloud under time pressure—report higher feelings of energy, creativity and power.[10]

One theory behind why we experience an energy surge with increased thought speed is that more dopamine stimulation occurs in our brains. Dopamine is a major chemical involved in transmitting brain signals. Whether or not this is the precise biological mechanism, it's likely that any activity that gets us to think fast may at least give us a temporary energy boost when we are feeling a slight low. This doesn't necessarily mean that thinking fast is a good long-term solution, but in the short term when you need to pick yourself up, it may be a good strategy. Try working on a crossword puzzle or Sudoku game under a stop clock for a quick boost of energy.

A caffeine boost

Coffee is one of the quickest, easiest and most popular natural energy boosts. Statistics show that more than half the population consumes it on a daily basis. You may have heard contradictory things from different sources regarding whether or not coffee is good for us. In actuality, this issue has been researched many times, and the general scientific consensus is that coffee in moderation is okay and a good potential stimulant. Used in this way, it shouldn't do you any harm. But the key word here is *moderation*. One or two cups a day is probably fine, and shouldn't produce any harmful effects. Some people prefer mornings, others afternoons or early evenings, depending on your own needs.

Energy drinks are also common nowadays, promising a rapid energizing effect, some claiming to last for several hours. Market research estimates that we spend billions of dollars annually on such products. But be very careful with these. As well as being unnaturally high in caffeine, many of them are also very high in sugar, which we have already learned is not a good solution. They have become especially popular among college students, and I have to confess I was an occasional offender myself when I had to be up late studying for those never-ending exams. But a major problem is that the high caffeine content (sometimes over 200 milligrams, compared to under 100 milligrams in a cup of coffee), can cause large fluid losses and potentially leave you severely dehydrated, especially as they are usually consumed in large amounts at a time, unlike coffee which is sipped slowly. Energy drinks are purposely designed to produce that sudden sugar high for maximal effect. But it's certainly not healthy to rely on these for an energy boost.

Taking breaks

We are not machines. While we obviously want to maintain high vigor and stamina, remember, too, that you are only human and need to recharge yourself from the constant hustle. It's vitally important that you take regular breaks in order to rest and re-energize. This is especially true during an intense workday. In fact, we as a society have worked the concept of a "rest" into all of our endeavors, from breaks during a sports game, to intermissions during a performance. This is for good reason. It's not natural to be able to keep your brain going at high energy for long periods of time without some respite. In one study from Louisiana State University, three different work-rest schedules were compared in people who worked at a computer screen.[11] The first group did an hour of work followed by a 10-minute rest, the second did 30 minutes of work followed by a 5-minute rest, and the third group took four shorter breaks in each hour followed by a 14-minute break after two hours. The participants were then asked to perform cognitive tasks such as addition and subtraction, and had to enter numeric data onto a computer. The results showed that the third schedule was much better for the workers in terms of reported levels of neck, back, arm, eyestrain, speed, accuracy and performance for both tasks. This frequent break strategy was therefore preferable to the longer rest schedules for fighting fatigue and subsequently increasing productivity. Although this was only a small study, the science behind the findings makes sense. Many authorities now advocate taking regular shorter breaks as a means of combating work fatigue and increasing overall output. No matter how behind or swamped you feel, keep this in mind. For your own good, you need to take regular breaks.

Back again to exercise

Unsurprisingly, being inactive is associated with feelings of fatigue. We've all been in a situation over the weekend where we find ourselves lazing around our house, devoid of all energy. The effect of exercise on mood that we discussed earlier is also inextricably linked to feelings of energy. When those endorphins improve your mood, your energy levels naturally elevate too. The two go hand-in-hand. Researchers from the University of Georgia conducted a large review of 70 studies involving more than 6,800 people. Each study investigated the effects of exercise training on energy and fatigue.[12] The pooled results conclusively found that exercise was associated with improved scores of both measures. More interestingly, the authors also concluded that the size of this effect may be larger than with drug treatments (which may sound familiar to you as well by now). In an experiment from California State University, investigators tested whether simple walking had any effect on energy levels in a group of almost 40 volunteers who were studied over a three-week period.[13] All of them wore a pedometer every day, and each night they completed a questionnaire to assess their feelings of energy. When the researchers looked at the results, they discovered a clear relationship between the number of steps everyone took and their overall reported energy levels. The more they walked in a day, the *more* energy they experienced.

And what if you are faced with a choice between a sugar boost or some exercise? Which one will benefit you more? Another well-designed study from the same institution helped answer this question by getting a group of students to either consume a sugar snack or take a brisk 12-minute walk.[14] Their self-rated energy levels afterwards were consistently higher after the walk, regardless of the time of day. On the other hand, the candy snack produced an initial period of increased energy, followed one hour later by the inevitable crash. It also appeared to produce more subjective tension in the short-term.

You may have thought that the more you exert yourself, the more tired you will feel, but the opposite is actually true. Exercise makes us feel *more* energetic. So next time you're feeling an energy low, or find yourself craving some caffeine, try a quick brisk walk or run up the stairs instead. This may be a better boost than your cup of coffee. And bearing in mind that mood and energy levels go hand in hand, you'll likely feel better too!

Sleep:
Why you need a good nightly snooze

It may seem strange to emphasize the importance of sleep in a chapter on how to energize yourself, but not getting a healthy sleep is one of the main reasons why we feel tired during the day. Sleep is a crucial part of our daily routine. And exactly *why* do we sleep? Scientists are still debating the precise reason, but it's universal throughout the animal world. Sleep is the time to rest our conscious brains and allow our bodies time to recharge. To be at your best during the day, you have to be getting enough sleep at night.

Unfortunately, statistics show that people in Western societies are sleeping less and less, with fewer than half reporting getting a sound rest.[15] A large proportion of people are even at the point where they are physically impaired as a result, with loss of concentration and slower reaction times. It's been estimated that losing four hours of sleep is equivalent to having a blood alcohol level of up to 0.1 percent. For a lot of us with busy schedules and responsibilities, getting the ideal amount of sleep every night can seem almost impossible, but it's important that we don't neglect this area of our lives.

Aside from the most basic effect on our alertness and energy levels, lack of sleep has also been proven to have a number of other detrimental health effects. In one large study of more than 10,000 adults, researchers found that women who regularly slept less than five hours per night had *twice the odds* of high blood pressure compared with those sleeping at least seven hours.[16] Another study from Columbia University of more than 4,800 people who were followed for a decade showed a similar pattern, even after controlling for obesity and diabetes.[17] One potential mechanism behind this effect is that sleep deprivation can lead to activation of the sympathetic nervous system, which we will learn more about in the next chapter, producing hormonal changes that increase our blood pressure.

With regards to our emotional and mental well-being, a team from Australia investigating almost 20,000 young adults under the age of 25, found that shorter sleep duration was strongly associated with psychological distress.[18] More than 50 percent of participants reporting fewer than six hours of sleep per night had high levels of current psychological distress compared to about 25 percent of those sleeping eight to nine hours a night. Each hour less of sleep correlated with a *14 percent increased* risk of psychological distress. And I can hear you asking right away whether lack of sleep leads to psychological distress, or is it really vice versa—namely, are people with psychological distress just *less* likely to sleep well? The researchers designed part of their study to answer this, by getting follow-up data on close to 3,000 of the participants 12 to 18 months later. This revealed that people who reported no distress at baseline, but then slept less than five hours per night, had more than a *three times higher* risk for new onset psychological distress. Other research has backed up these findings, repeatedly showing insomnia to be associated with an increased likelihood of future psychological problems.[19,20]

So how much sleep is ideal for our health? Rather than just use the old mantra of "at least eight hours," let's look at what the actual science says. A combined British and Italian team conducted a massive review to investigate the relationship between sleep duration and health outcomes.[21] Sixteen studies were reviewed that included almost 1.4 million people from eight different countries, who were followed for up to 25 years. The results were a real eye opener (again, no pun intended). When all of the data was pooled together, a shorter sleep duration of less than 5 to 7 hours was associated with a *12 percent increased* mortality. But here is the other interesting finding—so was a *longer* sleep duration of greater than 8 to 9 hours, which showed a *30 percent increased* risk. The reason for the range across sleep durations was that all of the studies were different. Nevertheless the trend was obvious; what scientists call a "u-shaped curve." Too *little* sleep is bad, and too *much* sleep is also bad. There has to be a happy medium.

Another theory as to why getting too little sleep is so damaging is that it directly produces physiological changes that increase our appetite and caloric intake. This in turn increases the risk of obesity and all of the associated problems. One small study from Chicago even showed that dieters had significantly more difficulty losing weight if they slept less than six hours, and lost *55 percent less* fat than those who slept more.[22] Getting excessive sleep is generally less of a problem in society, and it's likely that many people who get too much sleep already have health problems. We all know that when we sleep too long we often end up feeling more tired and lethargic than we would have if we had risen at our usual time, so perhaps our body is firing us a warning signal not to be too lazy.

The advice then is to get a good sleep of between 6 to 8 hours every night. Find your own ideal amount, but don't go too far under or over this amount. To reap even more advantages in terms of your own body clock, sleep and wake at the same time on most days. If you work odd shift patterns, it's a little bit more difficult, but sticking to a broad pattern as much as you can is advisable. Try not to regularly break up your sleep, like sleeping in two different bursts during the day and night. Sleep at only one time, and sleep continuously. And if you have difficulty getting to sleep, there are lots of things you can try to make yourself feel more relaxed before bedtime—like taking a warm bath, reading or meditating. If you find that your head is on the pillow and you are simply unable to fall asleep, then get up and do something else for 10 minutes, like reading, before trying again. Ironically, the more energetic and packed your days are, the more positioned you will be for a restful sleep. Finally, don't let your room be too hot. For most people the ideal sleeping temperature is somewhere around 65 to 70F.

Getting into the energy zone

Perhaps the most common non-medical reason that people experience a downturn in their energy levels is a negative state of mind that we have a two-syllable word for. *Boredom*. If you have nothing to do or your mind is not fully engaged in an activity, you will always tend to experience a sapping of energy levels. Boredom and monotony will drain the life out of you. This is innate in all of us. Maybe this serves a purpose too, as an evolutionary "kick" mechanism that is the driving force behind getting us to do stuff! We all need to be occupied. When was the last time that you were so totally absorbed in something that you lost track of time? Were you ultra-busy at work, entertaining guests or just so completely captivated by that movie? We've all had that sensation, when time becomes meaningless because we are so engrossed and energized. In sports this is often called "being in the zone." Another term for it is being "in the flow." If you think back to the last time you experienced this, you likely didn't have any problem with energy levels, because your mind was elevated to a whole new plane. Finding something that gets you to this level is not easy, and realistically it's impossible to maintain this feeling permanently. But when we do experience being in the zone, it's a timely reminder of how keeping our mind focused can dramatically make us feel more energized. As a general rule, being in this state will usually mean that we are busy with something. In other words, the complete opposite of boredom.

There's the tale of a farmworker who went up to a local wise man and complained that during the winter season he would feel lethargic and get very frustrated for no apparent reason at all. He asked the wise man to help him, and was promptly told that he would have to carry a full pail of water to the next town and then walk back again without spilling a drop before the wise man would give him the answer to his problem. The farm worker obliged and took a couple of days to complete his task. The wise man asked him on his return whether he had felt bored and lethargic during his two-day task. "Why, not at all, I was concentrating too hard on not spilling any water," replied the farmworker. "Of course that's so. You are only bored and lethargic because you have nothing else to focus your mind upon!"

On a more serious note, as the famous proverb goes, *an idle mind is the devil's workshop*. People who have too much time on their hands often get into trouble and fall into mischief. This happens on a macro level too, and is one of the reasons why, if you look at world history, bad economic times with massive unemployment often produce the most appalling brutal movements and ideologies.

So if you are bored with life, find something to spruce it up a bit and give your mind more opportunities to be occupied and captivated. If you really cannot stand your job and can't stop clockwatching, then work on a plan to change careers. If you are bored in the evenings, then join a new club or society. Find something that you feel passionate about that will get you into that zone. As Thomas Jefferson said, "Determine never to be idle. No person will have occasion to complain of the want of time who never loses any. It is wonderful how much may be done if we are always doing." Now that's great advice from one our most famous founding fathers.

HIGH PERCENTAGE ENERGY WELLNESS STEPS

- Eat low-glycemic foods

    Eat fewer simple and refined carbohydrates, and more fiber and protein

- Get outdoors and in nature

    Enjoy fresh air whenever you can, preferably in the sun

- Even indoors surround yourself with natural elements

    Give your home and office a "natural make-over" with plants and flowers

- Try some quick thinking exercises

    Like a crossword puzzle, Sudoku game, or speed-reading

- Have a cup of coffee

    Caffeine in moderation is okay

- Avoid sugar boosts during the day

    Skip candy and high-energy drinks

- Take a break

    Incorporate briefer but more frequent breaks into your schedule

- Get a good night's sleep

    Aim for at least 6 to 8 hours

- Keep your mind as occupied as possible

    Get yourself "in the zone"

CHAPTER FIVE

STRESS WELLNESS: CALMING YOURSELF

Stress is a phenomenon most of us know very well. It's everywhere and gets in the way of our well-being. In today's world, there are so many things to get stressed about. Whether you become stressed at work after you suddenly get given an unexpected task, when that certain person talks to you inappropriately, when your plan goes completely wrong, or when your son or daughter tells you that he or she is planning that solo trip to a dangerous part of the world, the physiological processes that lead to stress are all the same. The list of modern- day things to worry about is endless. Some of these we know are relatively minor issues, and others are much more distressing. Obviously a major shock or trauma in our lives is understandably going to make us feel stressed and upset. But there are so many other smaller things, which are probably not worth raising our blood pressure over for a minute longer than we need to.

The dictionary defines stress as "a specific response by the body to a stimulus, which disturbs our normal physiological equilibrium." That essentially sums it up. We are at a certain point where our natural balance is disturbed, and from then on stress and worry overtake our thought process. We can become totally consumed and lose our ability to see the overall picture. It's the difference in our minds between *what is* and *what ought to be*.

Although stress is mostly bad, remember that it isn't completely without purpose. Nobody is advocating that a stress-free life is achievable, or even desirable. One could make the argument that no human achievement would be possible if we were all wandering around in a state of eternal bliss feeling like we were in Shangri-La! We all need some stress to a certain extent to function, drive us forward and accomplish goals. But more about that later. What we need to do is learn to lessen the intensity of the feeling, channel it and transform it into a positive force that helps us solve our everyday problems.

A modern-day epidemic

There is a good reason why they call stress a modern-day epidemic. According to statistics[1-4], a majority of people regularly experience what they describe as moderate to high levels of stress, serious enough for them to be concerned about. Almost 75 percent report psychological and physical symptoms as a result. A large number of employees, 65 percent, say that work stress is causing difficulties, and 30 percent have yelled at a colleague. Sadly, over one in ten admits calling in sick, and one in five has quit a job because of stress. Even when we get into our beds at the end of the day, more than 40 percent report difficulty sleeping because they feel too stressed. Worse still, the time at which it hits us in life is now getting earlier and earlier, with stress levels soaring among high school and college students. These statistics all point to one simple fact. *We are a stressed-out society.*

As well as the pure economic cost, estimated at $300 billion a year[5] (which is greater than the entire GDP of Ireland), more important is the terrible strain on our bodies. Feeling stressed produces a number of changes that can lead to weak concentration, poor memory retention, uncharacteristic errors, difficulty sleeping, loss of appetite, performance dip, anger, emotional outbursts, and at its worst, alcohol or drug abuse. We've all been in a situation where some of these may have affected us. These negative reactions will then lead to more stress and a vicious circle of worsening symptoms that increases our chances of suffering anxiety, depression and other health problems.

I am often asked by my patients if stress could be contributing to their symptoms and illness. I always tell them that even if no controlled studies have been done to address the specific link of stress to their problem, it's highly likely that the answer is a strong *yes*. It goes without saying that during times of stress we are more prone to picking up almost any illness. That may not mean that it's the sole cause, but it certainly couldn't be doing anything other than running the body down.

The funny thing is that today we actually have so much *less* to be stressed about compared to any of our historical ancestors. We are not constantly looking for our next meal, we can stay warm in the winter, and we are not besieged by infections and plagues that used to ravage whole civilizations. In reality, we have it more comfortable now than ever before!

What we get stressed about

Here's a list of some common everyday stressors:

· Time constraints. Whether it is waiting in traffic or our desire to finish all our tasks by the evening, we feel under constant time pressure.

· Responsibilities. We are burdened by too many responsibilities and feel overwhelmed.

· Family. We feel stressed about our relationships with our spouse, parents, children and siblings. Relationships are not as we wish them to be.

· Unpleasant interactions. Even the briefest negative interaction can ruin our day.

· Career. We either feel bored in our jobs, not utilized correctly, overworked, underpaid or not making our way up the career ladder of success.

· School. Tests, assignments, coursework and more tests. It never ends.

· Finances. We can't balance the books. Outgoing is more than incoming and our lifestyle desires don't match our bank account balance.

· Unexpected bumps in the road. You had a path mapped out in your head about how something would work out and it's not entirely as you expected.

The biology of stress

In the early 20th century, Dr. Walter Cannon's pioneering research at Harvard Medical School led to him to coin the phrase "fight or flight" to describe the body's stress response. During times of perceived stress, all animals respond in a similar way when the sympathetic nervous system starts to fire. Heart rate and blood pressure increase, we start to sweat, and our pupils dilate as our vision and hearing become more acute. More importantly for us, we feel on edge, irritable and lose our ability to think straight. Our brain is getting primed for an emergency, and logical contemplative thinking takes a back seat. We become true animals again and can only think in black and white. When we are chronically stressed, this response is happening at a constant low level, impairing our ability to perform.

And here lies the irony about the stress response. The "fight or flight" reaction from the evolutionary standpoint has evolved as an emergency response to an imminently life-threatening situation. We are facing down a predator that wants to attack us, and we must act immediately, so our senses become more acute. Either we stand up and direct all our energies into fighting, or we channel them in the opposite direction and make a quick run for it (I know which one I would do if faced with a wooly mammoth). This reaction was never intended for worrying about our bank account, shopping list or sports team. That's the difference between us and other animals, who only reserve "fight or flight" stress for potential life or death situations, and experience it as a short, transient state of mind before moving onto their next goal. We, however, hold onto stress for much lesser issues and let things linger, experiencing a harmful chronic stress response.

The detrimental health effects

It has been known for centuries that stress adversely affects our health, but only recently have scientific studies actually proved that this is more than just common folklore. Not only does stress negatively impact our neurological and emotional capabilities, but it also impacts our cardiovascular system. It can even affect us superficially. Look at any before and after picture of US presidents to see the marked aging effects that such a stressful, high-profile job can have after four or eight years...well beyond the average superficial aging in that time.

In addition to adrenaline, another hormone closely linked to the stress response is *cortisol*, which is also naturally secreted by the adrenal glands in differing quantities during the day. When our bodies are under stress, both the adrenaline and cortisol levels shoot up. Research has shown that having high circulating levels of cortisol is potentially very harmful to us. One study from Holland followed more than 850 people over the age of 65 for six years after their urine cortisol levels were measured.[6] When the investigators corrected for other factors, they found that the people with the highest cortisol levels were a staggering *five times more likely* to suffer cardiovascular mortality.

Alarmingly, other evidence shows that stress can even directly reshape our brains. In a groundbreaking experiment from the University of California- Irvine, this effect was investigated on a group of laboratory mice that were exposed to stress for several hours in the form of loud music.[7] Afterwards, the mice underwent MRI scans of the brain. Amazingly, the mice that were exposed to this stress for just a few hours showed evidence of reduced numbers of neurons, the fibers that carry electrical signals in our brains. The researchers concluded that these changes may account for why people have difficulty with memory and retaining information when they are under acute stress. We all know from our own lives that this is true. Ever found that you forget routine simple things when you feel on edge?

One area of the brain that is directly affected by stress is the *amygdala*, which has become one of the most researched parts of the brain in recent years, something of a buzzword in psychology circles. The amygdala plays a major role in controlling our emotions. It is part of something known as the *limbic system*, which also includes two other important brain structures—the *hippocampus* and the *hypothalamus*. One study conducted at Cornell University investigated a somewhat tragic topic, the effects on the brain of children who had experienced prolonged rearing in orphanages.[8] The researchers looked at almost 80 children who were either reared partly in an orphanage, or brought up in a regular home environment. MRI scans were used to image the brain for any differences between the children. When the images were analyzed, it was found that children who were adopted later—in other words, had spent more time in an orphanage—had significantly *larger* adjusted amygdala volumes when compared to the other children. This effect was likely a direct response to the stress associated with being in an institutionalized environment, and is in line with other research that has shown larger amygdala volumes in stressed and anxious individuals. In fact, the phenomenon of our brains changing shape according to our external circumstances, experiences and emotions has a name in neuroscience. It's known as *neural plasticity*.

So remember that stress not only affects your brain, but can also *reshape* it in a negative way. If you have prolonged stress in your life, you need to change things fast. It's absolutely vital to your well-being.

The first step: Identify the problem

Go through the list of stressors earlier in this chapter and work out which ones apply to you. Likely a lot of them apply to you in differing proportions at different times. Like any problem, just being aware of the source of your stress and recognizing it is the first step towards solving it. Make a list of the five things that stress you out the most in your day-to-day life. Next, work out what your own unique stress reaction is when that adrenaline and cortisol starts to flow. Do you become irritable, wound-up or verbally uncontrolled? Flustered or angry? Do you despair or feel down? Have difficulty sleeping? Everyone is different. One person may have certain hot button areas of life that really lead to a lot of stress, while another person who, on the surface, appears to have a very similar life, may not get so stressed over exactly the same issues. Remember, the aim is not to avoid the stress completely, which is impossible, but rather to channel that energy into a more constructive force.

Whatever your issue is, when it hits, the stress hormones begin to flow. Your innate natural reaction starts to brew and you get ready to take aim and react. If you want to avoid that basic animal response, the first step is to gain back control over yourself and take a mental step back. It's a hard thing to do and requires much discipline and practice. We always feel worked up and flustered during those first few seconds, it's totally natural, and would probably be *unnatural* not to react that way. It's just a question of letting those hormones settle down in order for you to respond more logically and effectively. The angry, emotional response is usually something we regret afterwards. Reacting at that time is like trying to put out a fire with gasoline. For example, I have a self-imposed policy now, borne out of painful experience, that I don't respond to any work email that gets me flustered or worked up, for at least a few hours. If necessary, I draft it and keep it saved, but I won't send it for a while! The immediate response is always ill-thought out, emotional and counterproductive.

Meditation

When we use the word meditation, we are not necessarily talking about sitting cross-legged in a yoga position under a lotus tree. Meditation can also mean the simple act of mentally withdrawing for a little while and working out what to do next. This doesn't imply that you should be passive or not stand up for yourself. It simply involves taking a moment and composing yourself, while you work out the next step and hopefully avoid the detrimental effects of those stress hormones on your body. Looking at it logically, what's the point of working yourself up over getting stuck in a traffic jam? You are still stuck in it whether you are on edge or calmly listening to music. What's the point of stressing over that cancelled flight or train ticket? Either make alternative arrangements, or just work out the next step. Sure, you will be upset when things go wrong, but let it be for the least amount of time possible.

The physical act of the mental time-out can occur in different ways. Each one promotes a process called *mindfulness*. Mindfulness is a concept that has actually been around for thousands of years, and first started to widely surface in ancient Hindu and Buddhist philosophy. It involves a calm and serene awareness of the body's feelings. You are conscious of yourself and your surroundings. Nothing else is going on in your mind and you are not racing ahead with thoughts or worrying. It is the basis of all meditation techniques. Even for several seconds, practicing it can produce wonders in how you respond to a situation. Let's take an example. You see or hear about something that really fires you up. Your natural response is to follow that inner animal and immediately respond, often as we said, saying or doing something you might regret. Instead, close your eyes and take a few deep breaths, focusing on nothing except your own breathing. Breathe in and out, in and out. Enable more air to get into your lungs. Don't let your mind wander. Just be aware of your own senses and feelings. The longer the better, and the more effective your response will be. Just as important, you give your body time to counteract the effects of the stress hormones and return back to some kind of baseline. This works equally well with almost any situation, like when you suddenly turn onto that road which is full of traffic when you need to get somewhere fast (although this time, if you are driving, please don't close your eyes!). If you are face-to-face with somebody or in a group, obviously it may look somewhat strange if you start meditating like this, but you always have other options—like slipping away for a few minutes—while you calm yourself. This simple act of taking a short mental time-out and meditating can profoundly neutralize those stress hormones and help you to formulate a more desirable solution. Try it next time you feel stressed or overwhelmed.

If you are able to practice the art of meditation for longer periods, then it's likely to be even better for you. Incorporating a regular amount of meditation into your routine has proven benefits. In one study from China, researchers looked at the effect of meditation on stress and attention.[9] Students were divided into two groups, with 40 students given five days of meditation and mindfulness training (20 minutes each day), some of which was from ancient Chinese techniques, and the other acting as a control group. The students were then given some tasks to perform, with stress being induced by mental arithmetic problems. The results showed that the students who received meditation training experienced *less cortisol release*, and therefore, a lower stress response. Other studies have shown that practicing regular meditation can effectively reduce stress-related symptoms such as anxiety, depression and even chronic pain with long-lasting effects if the practice is continued.[10,11] In a Swiss experiment, researchers took 150 patients with the devastating neurological condition multiple sclerosis and gave half an 8-week program of mindful meditation training.[12] The techniques included deep breathing exercises and tasks that encouraged participants to focus on the present moment, rather than the terrible nature of their illness. The researchers assessed quality of life scores, depression and fatigue levels in all participants for six months. The results were impressive. The group that undertook the mindfulness training had significantly improved scores in most areas, even six months later. This was in spite of their actual illnesses staying the same.

At the most basic level, meditation is a mental time-out that helps you clear your mind, experience your senses and focus on the present moment. If you practice it more habitually, perhaps joining a yoga or tai-chi club, the improvements to your stress symptoms will likely be even more substantial. It's just about taking your brain away from all those worries and neutralizing the hormones.

Getting away from it all

One of the biggest beliefs in the Western world is in the ability of a nice vacation to help us de-stress every now and again. We've all heard about how a good time away is supposed to help recharge our batteries and enable us to come back feeling refreshed. It's conventional wisdom, but what does research say about whether vacations are good for us or not? The results may surprise you. In another study from Holland, researchers looked into the effects of a vacation on our baseline stress and mood levels.[13] More than 1,500 adults were surveyed, with two-thirds of them taking a vacation. Using questionnaires to assess perceived happiness and stress levels, it was found that the largest mood boost actually came *before* the vacation—from the simple act of planning it! Looking forward to a vacation was found to make people feel better for up to eight weeks. The bad news was that after a vacation, most participants quickly returned to baseline. Fascinatingly, the amount of stress experienced on the trip went on to influence post-vacation happiness. People who described their vacation as "stressful" or "neutral" did not have any post-trip happiness. People who said their vacation was "very relaxed" were the only people who experienced an increase in happiness after the trip, lasting only about two weeks. The length of vacation was not found to be particularly influential. The researchers concluded that planning a holiday seemed to be the most exciting part for the majority of people, and only those who reported feeling very relaxed during their trip had evidence of a post-trip mood and happiness boost. Reasons for a stressful vacation included disagreements with family or friends, and illness. Complaints on reaching home included the stress of an increased workload upon returning to the regular routine.

These findings have been replicated elsewhere, with other research confirming a similar pattern. One study from Israel looked specifically at the effect of vacations on job stress and burnout.[14] Almost 80 workers were studied before and after vacations, and the results showed that although they felt better during their vacation, they were back to experiencing burnout as soon as three days after returning to work. Like the Dutch study, people who were most satisfied with their vacations experienced the greatest stress relief.

So what insights can we draw from research like this? Intuitively, we probably already know from our own experiences that anticipating and planning a trip is exciting, but coming back from vacation is often a low when we return again to that huge workload. There may be no way around this "crash" effect upon returning to reality (unless you are sad enough to take your Blackberry with you on vacation!), but we can definitely try to make the most of things by keeping in mind a few points. First, rather than taking only one long vacation, plan shorter but more frequent vacations throughout the year if you are able to do so. Even weekend breaks can be great. Second, to experience the biggest boost from your trip, do everything you can to make sure that it involves the least possible stress while you are away. Plan your trip as much as possible and avoid any potential situations or company that you know will have you on edge. Are there any other little things you can do to increase your own enjoyment? If you have young children, look for any activities they can get on with in a safe place while you go and enjoy that relaxing theatre performance one evening. If you are going to a theme park, avoid going at a time when you have to stand in long lines in the sapping heat of summer—something not relaxing at all. Do you really *have* to go on that vacation with your extended family if you know it will not make you feel relaxed? Perhaps you could plan another trip with them instead. Vacations can certainly help reduce stress temporarily while you are away, but make sure you do everything possible to make it a tranquil time. And don't be surprised if one of the best parts is the excitement before you leave!

Spend time with a furry friend

Those of us who are animal lovers already know how much pleasure it is to have a cat or a dog. Our little furry friends never fail to make us feel better after a tough day. In fact, some of the most interesting research in the area of stress has looked into the curious ability of an animal companion to help us relax. In one well-designed study from the State University of New York, researchers evaluated the effect of pet ownership on blood pressure response to mental stress before and during treatment with a common blood pressure medication.[15] The study involved almost 50 volunteers who all had high blood pressure and reported a high-stress occupation. They were divided into two groups, both receiving the same blood pressure pill, but half were also required to get a pet dog or cat (let your doctor present you with that next time you are in his or her office). Of course, all the participants had previously consented to get the pet if assigned to that group, so it was not a complete surprise to them. Six months passed and then everyone was brought back to the office to be given a controlled mental stressor such as an arithmetic test, which was designed to induce a cardiovascular response. Bear in mind that both groups were given exactly the same blood pressure medication. Remarkably, the group assigned to pet ownership had significantly lower responses to mental stress, with heart rate and blood pressure responses at least *10 points lower*. The authors concluded that pet ownership blunted the blood pressure response to stress much more than the medication alone. From a medical standpoint, few medications have ever been shown to reduce blood pressure responses to stress, which makes this study result even more astonishing.

In a further, somewhat humorous, experiment from the same university, researchers compared the effects of friends, spouses and pets on cardiovascular response to stress.[16] Almost 250 married couples were studied, with approximately half owning a pet. Response to stress, this time either being mental arithmetic or immersion of a hand in cold water, was measured in their home environment. The participants were divided up in groups with either their spouse, friend, pet or none of the above. Again, the results were very interesting. The numbers showed that those people who owned pets had significantly smaller blood pressure and pulse responses to the stressful activities, as well as faster recoveries back to their baseline. The funny part of this study is that the biggest blood pressure responses—in other words, the most stressful responses—were found to occur in the presence of spouses!

The benefits of pet ownership may even extend to helping you recover from illness. In another well-known study, investigators looked at one-year survival rates of people who had suffered a coronary event.[17] More than 400 patients were studied, and all received baseline questionnaires to assess their psychosocial status. After one year, all were contacted again, and it was found that those with pets were much more likely to still be alive compared to the others, and this effect was *independent* of heart attack severity and any other psychosocial factors. Dog owners fared especially well. Whether this was due to differences brought about with physical activity or outside interactions was debatable, but the result was still clear. Moreover, as we age, the benefits may be even greater. Elderly people with pets have been found to make fewer visits to their physician[18], with dogs in particular appearing to provide a buffer in terms of stressful events that lead to physician contact, and to have less deterioration in their daily level of functioning compared to non-pet owners.[19]

And finally, how about pets at work? A survey from Eastern Kentucky University evaluated the effects on employees who were allowed to bring their pets to work.[20] Almost 200 employees from 31 companies completed anonymous questionnaires. The results conclusively showed that employees perceived pets in the workplace to reduce stress and positively affect employee health, especially obvious among people who already owned pets at home. Before all the animal lovers get too excited, this is obviously not going to happen in most organizations, and I can imagine the shock on my patients' faces if I walked into their rooms with my dog behind me!

All this evidence points in only one direction. Pets—especially, as most of the research has focused on, cats and dogs—are very good for us. When I was very young I remember my dad telling me that whenever I was having a bad day at school, I should just think of our two cats to help me feel better. While my dad has no background in psychosocial research, the premise of the advice was true. Pets are a very positive stress-reducing force in our lives. And just how do our furry friends do this? It's likely to be a combination of factors, including the sense of responsibility or dependence that they exert on us and the improved physical activity of dog ownership. Our relationship to animals is also relatively one-sided from an emotional standpoint, unlike our human relationships which can be a great source of stress. One survey found that almost half of respondents believe they know exactly what their pet is thinking and that their dog is far more likely to notice when they've had a bad day than their best human friend.[21] It's very difficult for a pet to really upset us. I know when I'm at home sometimes just seeing my dog or cat walk into the room helps me instantly feel less stressed and happier. They are wonderful beings that can really enrich our lives.

All that being said, remember as the saying goes, *a dog is for life and not just for Christmas*. If you're going to get a pet, be prepared for the enormous responsibility that goes with it. If you already have a pet, you are in the majority. According to the Census Bureau, almost 6 out of 10 US households own a pet, with the majority of these being dogs.

Relaxing foods, drinks and books

Tea is one of the most ancient drinks known to man, and we've already talked a little bit about its great health benefits in the first chapter. Tea has been used for centuries to help relieve stress, but only now have scientists actually studied this properly. A team from the United Kingdom took 75 healthy men and withdrew them from tea or other caffeinated beverages for four weeks.[22] At the beginning of the study, each participant underwent assessments of their blood pressure, pulse and cortisol levels, and also gave subjective descriptions of stress. They were then divided into two groups. The first group continued drinking a tea mixture made up of the same constituents as an average cup of black tea, and the other half were given a placebo treatment that looked and tasted the same way, but did not contain any active tea ingredients. Everyone was then exposed to a simulated stressful situation, as the researchers measured their cardiovascular and stress responses. The results showed that the active tea drinkers had significantly lower cortisol levels, *dropping by almost 50 percent* in the tea-drinking group compared with half as much in the placebo group. There was also an increase in subjective relaxation almost one hour after the task. The scientists concluded that these results signified a definite de-stressing effect of drinking tea. So switch the kettle on, and make yourself a cup of tea to help you relax. If we're talking green tea, it's packed with anti-oxidants too.

Let us return again to walnuts. In addition to the great cardiovascular benefits, an experiment from Pennsylvania State University looked at the effects of walnuts and walnut oil on the body's response to stress.[23] Researchers took 22 adults with elevated LDL "bad" cholesterol, and placed them on three different diets. The first diet contained no nuts, representing the typical American diet. The second contained about nine whole walnuts with a tablespoon of walnut oil per day, and the third was similar to the second but also contained flaxseed oil. All diets were matched for calories. After six weeks, all of the participants' had their stress response tested, and it was found that those who consumed the walnuts had significantly *lower* diastolic blood pressures in response to stress. This result is entirely plausible. It makes sense biologically and physiologically that good heart foods are also going to be beneficial for your stress reaction too, since the response is mediated by the cardiovascular system.

Finally, many people routinely pick up a book when they want to relax. Many use it as a sleep aid, as we've already discussed. As well as the obvious educational benefits of reading, research actually proves this technique can have a profound calming effect. One study showed that when a group of volunteers was exposed to various stressors, reading afterwards helped to reduce stress levels by almost *70 percent*.[24] Only six minutes of reading was needed to slow down the heart rate and ease muscle tension. This effect was found to be even better than listening to music. The researchers theorized that the relaxation occurred because our brains are forced to concentrate during reading. If we are enjoying a good book, our minds will escape the stress, helping our bodies return to baseline.

And back again to exercise

Do you notice how we keep returning to this? With its mood-enhancing and energizing effects, exercise is naturally going to be an excellent stress reducer too. One team from the University of Buffalo investigated this phenomenon in a group of 40 schoolchildren between the ages of 10 and 14.[25] The first group of students sat in chairs and watched a slideshow that depicted a journey to school.

The second group walked on a treadmill and watched the same slideshow. Afterwards, the children were exposed to a cognitive stressor and had their stress levels assessed. The results revealed that the group of children who had been walking experienced significantly *lower* levels of perceived stress compared to the stationary group, as well as lower pulse and blood pressure responses. Imagine then, if children—who are generally more resilient and less stressed than adults—could experience such an improvement after they walked, how much potential benefit an adult could get.

If you suddenly feel overwhelmed with stress one day and feel like you could explode, go for a quick walk or run. You can even take deep breaths and make it a meditation exercise too. Many people consider their post-workday gym session to be part of their daily stress therapy, and it's easy to see why.

Relaxing more in your life

From meditation to drinking tea, all stress-management techniques are acting in a similar physiological way. It's all just about reducing those stress hormones and letting your cardiovascular system settle down. There are things in life that are simply not in your control. Things like the weather, the horrible news report from the other side of the world, or even your favorite sports team losing. Take them for what they are. You will naturally feel frustrated and upset if it bothers you, but when it's something you really cannot control, try to get it out of your mind as soon as possible. It's unconstructive to focus so much on uncontrollable things. The television news, in particular, can be distressing and give you a terribly skewed picture of the world. I think newscasters should be mandated to report good news as well!

If you find yourself with thoughts and worries racing through your mind and feel stuck in a stressful situation, try writing down your concerns and see if you can come up with any solutions. Conflict is an inevitable part of life. It's impossible to completely avoid it. Once you accept that conflict is something that can exist in any situation—with a customer sales rep, a work colleague or even a friend—it's a start to feeling more philosophical about it. Let the conflict hit your emotions, think about it and then take a step back and consider the problem from a logical viewpoint.

There are actually vast opportunities in many of our perceived everyday stressful situations. Take that traffic jam when you're at a standstill. Use your time wisely. Do you have friends you need to catch up with? Make that call on your hands-free! Have you longed for some quiet thinking time all day? Now's your chance. If a work project turns out to be a disaster, then what can you learn from it to make tomorrow better? We can all change our own attitude towards how we look at things. If we are inflexible and rigid, then this will not only cause us stress when things don't work out as we want, but will also make us miserable too. It helps to be pragmatic.

Sometimes we simply have to say *no* to avoid all those extras in life that are an unnecessary added burden. If you don't need to take on that additional task because of your already overloaded schedule and time constraints, then don't. If your week is already packed, then do you really need to promise a friend that you will make that long trip to visit them, or do a favor for a work colleague that you just don't have time to do? Save it for the next time. Try not to overload your to-do list to the point where you've only made yourself feel tense. There are only a certain number of minutes in a day.

Overanalyzing situations and overreacting is another surefire way to keep on feeling uptight. Having talked about pets, we can learn a lot from them in this respect. Watch what happens when a dog doesn't get what it wants. It might sulk for a while, but invariably regains its baseline when another challenge or opportunity is placed in front of it. Animals know how to move on much better than we do, and they certainly don't waste time dwelling on negative emotions. If you have something that is weighing on your mind, try to get into the habit of either dealing with it or finding something else to focus your energies on. Holding onto problems can really wear us out.

Finally, remember that a life without stress and complications is not realistic. Expecting and anticipating problems makes handling them so much easier. When you take on a challenging task, know that problems will come up. If something does go completely according to plan, then more power to you. Enjoy it and savor the moment. In fact, if you prepare yourself for hitches and none happen, it's something to feel even better about! A lot of our everyday stresses can be passed off as a normal part of life. *C'est la vie*, as they say. Never allow something small to ruin your precious day. Just pick yourself right up again. So next time you feel those stress hormones brewing, simply take a step back and let those emotions subside. If you can, transform them into a positive force, and hopefully you will be able to cope a little better next time.

HIGH PERCENTAGE STRESS WELLNESS STEPS

- Identify and recognize your hot button issues

    Everyone has unique stressors

- Take a step back when stress hormones begin to flow

    Just allow a moment to let your cardiovascular system settle down

- Regularly meditate and practice deep breathing

    Do this alone or in a group setting

- Plan as many vacations as possible

    Shorter, but more often, is better

- Consider getting a pet

    A dog or cat can do wonders for relieving stress

- Drink tea regularly

    Switch on the kettle and pour yourself a cup

- Read more books

    Escape to another world

- Many stresses are a normal part of life

    Conflict is inevitable and certain issues are simply not in your control

CHAPTER SIX

SOCIAL WELLNESS: YOUR DAILY INTERACTIONS

Several years ago, former President Bill Clinton addressed a Labour Party conference in the United Kingdom. He began reminiscing on his time as President, and how one of the high points had been when scientists announced that they had successfully decoded and sequenced the entire human genome. He said that what he found particularly interesting was that when the scientists looked closely at the genetic sequence, they found that essentially all human beings were 99.9 percent identical, and that the difference within any given community was far greater than the differences between societies thousands of miles apart. In other words, if you were to take a group of people from South America and compare them to a group of people in an isolated country like Iceland, the genetic differences *within* those groups would be larger than the differences *between* the cultures. That's an incredible fact. Yet despite our being 99.9 percent the same genetically, most of us are frequently guilty of spending 99.9 percent of our time thinking about the 0.1 percent of us that is different from our fellow human beings! President Clinton concluded by saying that even if any of us suddenly got everything we ever wanted in making us richer, more successful or more beautiful than our neighbor, if we then found ourselves all alone in the world, it would not amount to a "hill of beans." How profound…and how very true.

As the famous 17th century poet John Donne wrote, *No man is an island*. We as humans are social animals who spend most of our lives interacting with other people. We are all defined by our relationships. How we go about these, and the positive or negative repercussions that result, will ultimately have a direct impact on our well-being. One of the greatest ironies of our physical make-up is that the tongue is built to be among the softest and most flexible muscles in our bodies, but on a day-to-day basis it is actually the most powerful. As we've seen from dealing with stress, even the briefest interaction can often have a dramatic effect on how our day is going. Good communication is key to healthy relationships with family, friends and colleagues.

It's also important to remember that we are communicating even when we are not talking. Have you ever seen somebody whose demeanor and expressions convey anger or sadness? They have not even said a word to you, and have already inadvertently announced their feelings to you. The same process is going on all the time with you. Your body language is constantly sending messages to other people. From our facial expressions, eyes, mouth, hand gestures and body posture, we are always talking to the outside world!

We are judgmental by nature

Think how often you meet a new person. Do you think you are nonjudgmental? The evidence would suggest otherwise. In fact, our brains are primed to make instantaneous judgments about people. In the third season of the hit television show "Britain's Got Talent," an unknown contestant stepped onto the stage in front of a packed studio audience. She was about to sing the famous song from "Les Miserables," "I Dreamed a Dream." Her name was Susan Boyle, and within a few days she would become a worldwide sensation. One of the reasons for the Susan Boyle phenomenon was that she took everyone by surprise. If you watch the video on YouTube, you will see that the audience and judges dismiss her chances before she even starts singing, based on her physical appearance and mannerisms. Many of them are shrugging, laughing and openly deriding her. This is a sad indictment of how quick we all are to judge people before we even give them a chance. On a more positive note, much of the conversation and media focus after her performance actually focused on this self-realization—that we are by nature prone to these quick and rash assessments of people. But at the same time, it's really something we can't help!

An interesting study from Princeton University looked into this very topic.[1] Researchers conducted five experiments, each focusing on a different trait: attractiveness, likeability, competence, trustworthiness and aggressiveness. It would logically follow that only attractiveness and perhaps aggressiveness should be snap judgments, with the others taking some time to size up. More than 100 undergraduate students were shown unfamiliar faces for either 100, 500 or 1000 milliseconds. That's one-tenth, one-half and one second. A very small timeframe, a blink of an eye. For each face, the students were asked to make a snap trait judgment and then to express their confidence in the judgment. Immediately after seeing the photo, a question would appear on the computer screen asking something like, "Is this person competent?" The researchers compared the participants' judgments to those made by a control group that did not have time constraints. The results were thought-provoking. Even after a tenth of a second exposure time, the trait judgments were very similar to those made in the absence of time constraints. This meant that an exposure time of just *100 milliseconds* was enough for people to make specific judgments about people for all five of the character traits. Conventional wisdom would suggest that more exposure to a face produced better judgments, but this wasn't so. Additional time to look at someone's face did not appear to make much difference, and if anything, actually produced more negative judgments. The only thing that did increase was the participants' own confidence in their judgment, which was particularly pronounced from 100 to 500 milliseconds. Another interesting finding was that the highest correlation between judgments made after 100 milliseconds and those made in the absence of time constraints was in the area of trustworthiness and not, as the authors thought, in attractiveness. This could be because from an evolutionary standpoint, quick detection of trustworthiness is necessary for survival and detecting potential danger. Even more remarkably, the scientists who conducted this study concluded that we may even be able to make judgments about people in *less* than a tenth of a second, but such a small timeframe would be extremely difficult to actually study in a controlled environment.

These findings have been backed up by other studies too. For instance, one experiment showed that a split-second judgment on photos can successfully predict the result of Congressional elections about 70 percent of the time, as people decided in a blink of an eye whom they did and didn't like, or whom they judged incompetent.[2] Another study from the University of Iowa looked at what effect a handshake has on peoples' perceptions of you.[3] You may think that a handshake is a relatively simple and non-consequential gesture. After all, it's been around for thousands of years, and believed to have originated as a way for two people to show that they have no weapons hidden from each other! But the *way* you do it is actually very important. The results from the Iowa study showed that people who start job interviews with a firm, strong handshake were always judged more favorably than those who have a softer, more limp handshake. Good hand-shakers were also viewed as more extroverted.

We are therefore processing information about new people faster than we could ever be aware of. What this highlights is two important points in our interactions with others. First, we should not always trust our immediate impressions, because they occur too fast to be based on well-thought logic. Our instincts may often be right, and this quick propensity to make judgments exists for a reason—to alert us to potential dangers— but at the same time they are often wrong, as in the case of Susan Boyle. Second, it also emphasizes just how important it is to try to make a good first impression with people. If you are going for a job interview, meeting a client, or encountering anyone else for the first time, those initial few milliseconds could make or break you.

Eyeing up

Making direct eye contact is the most basic first step in the communication process, and is universal throughout the animal kingdom. All of us have been able to recognize and identify eye contact since very early in our development. One team of scientists studied 17 three-day-old babies, and got them to sit on an adult's lap in front of a screen that showed pictures of people.[4] Two faces of the same person were flashed up. One of them looked directly forward, and the other looked away with their eyes. The results showed that newborns looked almost *70 percent longer* at the faces looking directly at them. And these were just three-day-old babies. Studies like this lead scientists to believe that the deep brain connections that are receptive to eye contact form when we are still in the uterus, before we are even born; this is not something that is learned from experience. In another experiment conducted in slightly older babies, the same researchers directly measured brain electrical activity in a group of 15 four-month-old infants. Again, the infants all sat on their parent's lap directly in front of a computer monitor. Their attention was drawn to the screen with a color cartoon. When they looked, faces were put up on the screen instead, with either direct or averted gaze. The testing revealed the amplitude of brain waves was higher in response to direct gaze than to averted gaze. Basically, the brain was stimulated more when the babies realized that they were being looked at!

The ability to look directly into the eyes and engage with people is therefore a primitive need, wired from our very beginnings. There is a saying that the *eyes are the window to the soul*. We need this contact to interact and assess the other person. Have you ever talked to someone who doesn't maintain eye contact when he or she speaks? You probably instantly got the impression that the person is disinterested or perhaps even untrustworthy. It's a natural instinct that tells us someone doesn't want to be there, or worse, has something to hide. I have encountered a few people myself, from salesmen to colleagues, who just don't make eye contact when they're talking to people. Interestingly, with some of my fellow physicians, I have heard negative feedback from patients and families regarding their interactions. I feel bad sometimes, because a lot of them are fine doctors, but the cold truth is that gaze avoidance is easily interpreted as indifference and evasiveness. Not good qualities, especially for a physician.

If you want to endear yourself to people, there is even evidence that looking directly at others makes them more liable to copy your movements, and in doing so, like you more! Two inspired researchers sought to determine what effect eye contact would have on imitation of hand movements.[5] In one experiment, 20 students watched a movie clip of an actress who made a head movement followed by a hand movement. The participants then had to respond as quickly as possible with their own hand movement as soon as the actress's hand moved. The video would either show the actress turning towards the camera, and giving direct eye contact, or conversely away from the camera. The participants' reaction time and hand movements were then recorded. The results were intriguing. When the movie clip showed the actress looking directly at the participant, the reaction times were consistently *faster* in inducing similar hand movements. The researchers concluded that direct gaze is a powerful social signal that can rapidly result in unconscious imitation. The reason why this is important? Well, many psychologists have shown that there is a close relationship between the unconscious imitation of other people's behaviors and the copier also liking the person. In psychology circles, this is known as the *chameleon effect*. Anything that makes people more likely to copy your behaviors increases the chances that you will get on well. Imitation really is *the sincerest form of flattery*. Could the same be true for decisions too? If you want people to do something, should you make an effort to meet them directly so that you can sit face-to-face and look them in the eye more? It makes absolute sense.

Hence, this most basic first step in communication is of the essence. We are all hard-wired to react to eye contact. Whether it's getting your child to clean their room, cutting that all-important work deal, persuading a colleague to do you a favor, or just wanting to get along with someone- look directly into their eyes.

Facial expressions

Our brains not only respond to direct gazes, but are also highly adept at recognizing and storing information about peoples' faces. This is why we often see facial likenesses in inanimate objects (see any of the many news stories of people identifying faces in random rock faces and food items). Consider this. You probably encounter thousands of different people every year, and form close associations with dozens of them. Your brain could pick out a familiar face in a split second. You can't do that with other objects which you also encounter thousands of times. You may see innumerable numbers of apples, trees, tables and doors every year, none of which is completely identical. Yet you cannot pick these out from one another. Faces are a very different proposition for your brain.

Once we have identified that new or old face, the expressions that arise from it are sending us signals all the time, something that again is a primal recognition process. Another study involving a group of 17 newborns with an average age of just two days found that they spent almost *25 percent more* time looking at a happy than a fearful face on a screen.[6] This not only provides evidence that our ability to distinguish facial expressions comes very early, but also shows that even newborns have a preference for happiness! Despite the multitude of different societies and cultures across the world, facial expressions are surprisingly universal. From an isolated jungle tribe to a high-tech Western society, we have an innate knack for being able to pick up what the person in front of us is feeling just from looking at his or her face. Researchers at the Universities of Virginia and California-Berkeley showed a group of 40 undergraduates in Wisconsin and a group of 40 people from rural India photos containing the same set of 14 facial expressions and asked them what happened to make the person feel that way.[7] Two different methods were used by the investigators to get responses. One involved a simple description of the faces and the other involved being asked to pick a word that described them. The results showed wide agreement in the faces that represented happiness, surprise, anger, disgust and embarrassment. This despite the societies being as far apart culturally and technologically as possible.

The power of your smile

Without doubt, the most powerful facial expression we have at our disposal is our *smile*. It follows popular logic that we smile only when we are happy and upbeat, but now research is in fact showing that the simple act of smiling can actually induce biological changes that can then go on to *make* us happy.[8,9] Put another way, smiling not only sends a powerful signal to those around you, but may also have a dramatic effect on your *own* feelings. On a basic communication level, smiling signals our intent to cooperate and show trust towards people. On a psychological level, it is picked up immediately by the other person.

In a combined American and British study, 120 volunteers were shown a series of photographs and then asked to rate the peoples' faces on a series of personality traits.[10] Their answers consistently showed that being rated as cooperative was related to the presence or absence of a smile. People who smiled were judged to be more cooperative, and those who didn't, less so. The second part of the study got a bit more interesting. This was designed to see how much people trusted a smiling versus a non-smiling counterpart in a game with financial stakes. Each participant was seated at a computer terminal and played a game whereby they had to cooperate with a perceived counterpart in order to win money on a video game. They were all shown a photo of this person first. The results showed that people trusted smiling photos in almost 70 percent of decisions, almost *25 percent more* than non-smiling photos. Thus, seeing the smile positively affected trust among strangers, since nobody knew their supposed counterpart beforehand. And when the results were analyzed even further, it was found that men were more influenced by smiling than women, and that men were more likely to trust women, and women more likely to trust men- when they smiled!

At the same time, it's not simply a question of just putting on a "happy face." Scientists actually distinguish between two types of smile, known as the *Duchenne* (named after the famous 19th-century French neurologist) and the *non-Duchenne* smiles. Anatomically, the

Duchenne smile involves the contraction of the zygomaticus major and orbicularis oculi muscles on your face. The ends of your mouth are raised and your eyes scrunch up. This is a true spontaneous smile that is very difficult to fake, and reflects genuine emotions and happiness. On the other hand, a non-Duchenne smile involves only the zygomaticus major muscle, and is easy to make voluntarily whenever you like, not necessarily being a reflection of your real emotions. Most of the time, when considering other peoples' reactions, a genuine smile is really the only one that will likely have an effect. A team of researchers from Finland investigated this by conducting an experiment into peoples' emotional reactions to smiling.[11] Their analysis showed that looking at a genuine smile induced feelings of pleasure and empathy, much more so than a fake smile. We can all probably relate to this, because it's quite easy to spot a bogus emotion a mile away. New research even shows that wearing a fake smile also makes people unhappy themselves! In an experiment from Michigan State University, a group of bus drivers was followed for two weeks.[12] Some were asked to put on a fake smile to their customers, and others were asked to display their smiles only after cultivating positive thoughts. Psychological tests found that the bus drivers who put on forced smiles experienced significantly *lower* moods and happiness levels. So non-genuine smiling doesn't do you, or others, any good.

Perhaps the most fascinating research of all into the effects of smiling involves the hypothesis that a smile can be a predictor of future life events. In a unique study from DePauw University in Indiana, investigators looked into the relationship between smiling in photos and divorce in later life.[13] The rationale behind being able to make such audacious predictions rests on a theory in psychology known as *thin-slicing*. This involves using the shortest of time periods to gain profound insights into someone's character and emotions. We've already read about how quick we are to make snap judgments, but thin-slicing uses scientific techniques to gain the insights, usually by behavioral patterns. In this case, facial smiles in photographs were used. The researchers tested their theories on a sample of more than 300 graduates, and looked back at their graduating yearbook photos using a scientific scale to measure smiles according to the use of facial muscles. These people were then contacted (bear in mind, this was decades after the photos) and asked to complete a questionnaire that inquired specifically about their marital life. The results were startling. There was a direct correlation between smile intensity, and whether or not participants were likely to divorce at some point in their lives. That is, the *less intense* they smiled, the *more likely* they were to divorce. This was true for both males and females. To expand the scope of their theory to see if it could apply to another population, the researchers then went on to test a random community sample of 55 middle-aged volunteers. They were all asked to send photos from the ages of 5 to 22, including school, family and wedding pictures, and then asked to provide details of their marital status. When the photos were analyzed using the same technique, the researchers found the *exact* same pattern. The more intense the smiles, the less likely they were to divorce. And what was the craziest thing about this part of the study? The average age of the people in these photos was just *10* years old! The investigators concluded that these findings could have been due entirely to the thin-slicing phenomenon. Namely, the photos reflected peoples' underlying emotional tendencies, which then influenced behavioral processes. A person who smiles more is likely to be more friendly, cooperative and outgoing, and the people they interact with may be more likely to mimic the same behaviors. In this way, having positive tendencies can result in more positive responses. Whatever the exact mechanism, it's easy to see how this type of emotional flow is likely to result in better relationships. This is of course all a very crude analysis and may sound a little far-fetched to some. Nevertheless, the results of the study were clear and equivocal. Smiling in photos somehow predicted a major life event like divorce.

And how about smiling for your own longevity? In another study, this one from Wayne State University, researchers looked at 230 photos of baseball players from the 1950s and analyzed the players' faces, from those without a smile, to those with a full Duchenne smile.[14] Those who smiled the most lived on average seven years, or almost *10 percent*, longer than the group with no smile!

Interestingly, if a smile is viewed as a sign of cooperation and trust, then traditional evolutionary science would argue that those who are cooperative or altruistic have a survival *disadvantage*. This is because at the most basic level in nature, animals that pursue their own self-interest typically have an advantage in getting what they want. This doesn't hold true though for humans. We do not live in the animal kingdom any longer, and for us there are great gains from being cooperative and trusting.

What does all of this mean practically? Of course, smiling is usually a reflection of your underlying state of mind. Happier people do smile more effortlessly anyway. As we've said, a fake smile is unlikely to get you anywhere, and indeed most of the research into smiling uses detailed profiles to distinguish between genuine and fake smiles. And unfortunately, for some people, smiling just doesn't come naturally. There are some notorious examples of famous people, many of them politicians, who just can't put on a natural smile. Gordon Brown, the former British Prime Minister, was an example, and there are some hilarious videos on the Internet of him attempting to smile. This is not necessarily a reflection of his underlying mood or competence—it's just what he is. But if you are able to do things or be in situations that make you genuinely smile more, then go ahead and do them. Whether it's your favorite hobby, enjoying yourself with friends, or watching a great comedy, smiling more in life is only going to be a good thing. Smiling and laughter really are among the best of medicines.

The importance of a compliment

There is a line from the hilarious British comedy series, "Only Fools and Horses," when Del Boy says to Rodney, *a compliment is the easiest thing to give and the nicest thing to receive.* While this pearl of wisdom may come from an unlikely source, what Del Boy says is true. Complimenting people brings about an immediate boost to the other person, and if you are on the receiving end, makes you feel good too. Now this isn't to say that you shouldn't be sincere, because like smiling, fakeness is picked up immediately. But if there is something worthy of a compliment, you should go ahead and do so.

Let's take an example from another unlikely source. One that could even earn people some more money too! Tipping behavior in restaurants. In a small but informative study, researchers looked at the effects of giving compliments on how much tipping waiters received.[15] The experiment involved two male and two female servers, all in their twenties, in four restaurants. The servers were told that after taking their customers' orders, they would either compliment the peoples' dinner choices or not. Before going to the tables, they would choose from a group of pennies to find out whether to give a compliment at any given table. More than 1,100 customers were studied, and after each table left, the tip was recorded. Researchers found a more than 3 percent *increase* in tipping behavior in the compliment group. This may not seem like very much, but considering that tips are generally under 20 percent, this difference is significant. But the researchers found something else that at first seems inexplicable. When the party size was larger, compliments were actually found to have a *negative* effect. The more the waiters complimented people in a large group, the fewer tips they would receive. These findings are important for several reasons. Looking narrowly at the restaurant industry, where servers are not entitled to minimum wages because of the belief that they will earn money in tips, a small difference like this could amount to hundreds of dollars a year. The discovery that complimenting had a negative effect on larger dining parties highlights the problem of insincerity. Complimenting every person at a crowded table comes across as such, so it's not really an effective thing to do, and certainly not endearing to the customer. The good news though for servers was that in the study, 70 percent of the tables were just two to three people.

These effects are applicable across other service jobs too. A similar experiment involving hairdressers yielded even more dramatic results.[16] Two hairdressers gave different levels of compliments to more than 100 customers. This time, the average tip was about 33 *percent higher* in the compliment group, when the hairdressers gave positive comments such as, "Your hair looks terrific!"

Did the people who gave higher tips do so because they felt good or because they liked the person more? Who knows, but the result was still the same. Research like this simply confirms the profound effects of giving a compliment on peoples' psyche. And all being said, by far the most important place to use compliments is in your *personal life*. This may be difficult to measure in controlled studies, but deep inside we all probably know from our own experiences the power of compliments, especially when it comes from someone who is important to us. So go ahead and compliment at every opportunity that deserves one. A family member who has worked hard. A friend who is dressed well. A colleague who has done a good job. There are dozens of everyday occasions worthy of a good compliment.

Apologies

It is only human to make mistakes. If we are at fault, apologizing is one of the most meaningful things we can do. According to a Canadian research survey, people apologize an average of four times a week.[17] However, the researchers found that there are vast differences in *whom* we are more likely to apologize. Almost 50 percent of apologies were to friends and only 7 percent to family. Even strangers fared better than family, receiving 22 percent of apologies. Whether you are male or female also plays a part. Intuition would (should) tell us that women apologize more readily than men. Another Canadian team looked into this very question.[18] In the first part of their study, 66 men and women kept a daily diary of all offenses they committed or experienced and whether or not they had apologized. The results showed that women did indeed offer more apologies than men, but also that they reported more offenses. In other words, women were offended much more often but, similarly, also offered more apologies for their own behavior. Crucially, there was *no* difference in the number of offenses it took to result in one apology. So men simply apologized less because they had a higher threshold of what an offense is. But they were still statistically just as likely to apologize when they believed they had done something wrong! In the second part of the study, 120 men and women were asked to evaluate both imaginary and recalled offenses such as being rude to a friend. The men again consistently rated the offenses as less severe than women did. These different ratings of severity obviously then predicted whether or not an apology was offered. I'm guessing this could be the subject of a whole other book. But the question this research really poses probably boils down to this. Are men *insensitive*? Or are women *too* sensitive? Either way, it's likely men and women will still be debating this in a thousand years time!

On the other side of the coin, it's important to graciously accept an apology when one is offered to you. The act of making amends and moving on is paramount in maintaining harmony in all personal relationships. Of course, the apology has to be real, but try not to hold onto those resentments and grudges.

When being a poser can be good for you

Aside from facial and rhetorical expressiveness, a large part of nonverbal communication includes body language, and in particular, your pose or posture. This not only reflects your feelings and level of comfort, but can also directly represent your power rank relative to another person or group. There have been fascinating documentaries that analyze how world leaders interact with each other, and what their body postures say about who the subordinate one is. But in one combined study from Columbia and Harvard Universities, researchers turned this theory on its head, and examined whether peoples' postures can actually *cause* power.[19] The researchers took 42 volunteers and randomly assigned them to perform either high- or low-power poses. To keep the participants in the dark about the nature of the experiment, they were not told about the true purpose of the test, and had an EKG machine attached to them while they were in the different poses. They adopted the two different postures for one minute each. The high-power poses included leaning back on a chair with hands behind their head and feet up on the table, or leaning forward with hands placed on the table. The low-power poses included sitting in a chair with hands crossed over between legs, or standing up with legs crossed and arms folded. These poses are based on the theories of maximal and minimum expansiveness and openness, which are postures widely adopted in the animal kingdom to express either power or submissiveness. The more you expand yourself, the more power you are emanating, and conversely, the smaller you make yourself, the more submissiveness you are expressing. What the researchers wanted to find out was whether temporarily adopting these positions would have an effect on the volunteers' biology and psyche. Saliva samples were taken before and after the poses to measure cortisol and testosterone levels. The hormone testosterone reflects status and dominance throughout the animal kingdom. The participants' risk-taking behavior was then measured with a gambling task, and a questionnaire assessed their feelings of power. The gambling task involved being given $2 and told they could either keep the money or roll a die and have a 50/50 chance of either doubling the money or losing it all. The results were dramatic. Participants who adopted high-power poses had a significant *increase* in their testosterone levels after the pose, compared with a *decrease* in testosterone following the low-power pose. When the cortisol results were analyzed, the opposite effect was found. The high-power poses resulted in a decrease in cortisol levels compared with the low-power poses. With the gambling test, the high-power posers were significantly more likely to focus on rewards and take the risk. More than 86 percent took the risk, compared to only 60 percent of the low-power posers. The questionnaires also revealed that the high-power posers reported feeling significantly more powerful and in charge!

Experiments like this show that our nonverbal behaviors are not merely a reflection of our underlying psyche—but can actually *influence* it. A simple brief pose in the volunteers was enough to induce significant changes in their physiology and psychology. This has significant implications for everyday life. Adopting a power pose may help you feel a heightened sense of self-confidence. Be careful though to match the pose with the situation. Sitting with your hands behind your head may not be a good idea for a job interview, for instance. On the other hand, if you consistently adopt poses based on minimal expansiveness, such as curling up or folding your arms, then this will not only reflect submissiveness or defensiveness, but can also make you more likely to feel that way.

Getting along

We all know someone who seems to have flourished purely because of their ability to get along with people. Right or wrong, it often appears that style triumphs over substance in our society. There are people who climb the career ladder more quickly, make the right connections, and generally get whatever they are after, whether it's at work, at home or even in a shop! Their success lies in their ability to *connect*.

In a study titled "Competent Jerks, Lovable Fools," researchers looked into what kind of people employees prefer to work with.[20] Conventional thinking would tell us that when people need help regarding a difficult task, they would pick the most competent colleague. It turns out it's not quite that simple. The participants, who were from a large variety of organizations, were asked how often they had worked with other people in the organization, and were then asked to rate the people in terms of likeability and competence. Amusingly, four different caricatures were produced. The *competent jerk*, the *lovable fool*, the *lovable star*, and finally, the *incompetent jerk*, who obviously has the least going for him or her! In total, data on more than 10,000 work relationships was collected from organizations as diverse as technology companies and luxury goods corporations. The results were surprising. No matter the type of company, everybody wanted to work with a lovable star. Okay, no shock there. But here's where things got interesting. You might expect that out of the other combinations, competence would triumph, especially with managers. But no. Personal feeling came strongly into play, and competence was almost irrelevant when people were strongly disliked. By contrast, those who were liked were sought out, whatever their level of competence. The take-home message was that in most settings competence alone is not enough. You need to get along with your peers as well. If you don't, you are much less likely to be perceived well, and probably won't have doors open to you that would otherwise enable you to reach your full potential.

This likeability factor applies even at the highest levels—possibly even more so. One of the reasons cited for George W. Bush's successful run against John Kerry in the 2004 presidential election was that he was judged to be much more likeable...someone "you could go out for a drink with." Other experiments have shown that during political televised debates, nonverbal hostile behavior displayed by candidates has a big impact on the audience. In one study, students viewed televised debates where they were watching the nonspeaking opponent's background reactions on a split screen.[21] The students watched four versions of the debate, and the results showed that the debater was perceived to be less appropriate when he displayed any background disagreement compared to when he did not. In these circumstances, the speaker was judged as most appropriate. People basically gravitated away from the non-amicable candidate. A similar effect was noted during one of the 2008 presidential debates, when John McCain's nonverbal background disagreements were viewed as hostile and unappealing by some analysts.

Over the years, I've heard many patients talk about "how nice a doctor is." On one level, this is an entirely nonsensical thing to say, because the only real concern should be whether that doctor is competent and can get you well again! But we can't escape our humanness and desire to form emotional connections. In fact, whether it's your doctor, lawyer, financial adviser or accountant, unless there is some huge deficiency in competence, most people would go for amiability rather than the bad communicator with a textbook recital on the tip of their tongue. I see this every day in medicine, with the scientific whiz kids often not endearing themselves to the patients they meet, but consistently able to ace their exams. It may be possible to overlook with a computer programmer or technician, but obviously becomes a significant problem in any job where it is necessary to spend significant amounts of time communicating with people.

It's not necessarily a choice either between style and substance. The two do not have to be mutually exclusive. Having both is always better! But being hostile or selfish to others will never take you as far as getting on with people and being generally likeable. And don't see this as bending, being weak, or not pursuing your own goals. It's just about mutual respect and teamwork. Inflexibility is a weakness, because *the tree with the most fruit always bends the most*.

Emotional intelligence

The term *emotional intelligence* is a relatively new concept, but has really been a cornerstone of our daily interactions since time immemorial. Traditionally, at least in scientific and academic circles, the main measure of someone's intelligence was always based on IQ.

Now, however, an individual's emotional intelligence is believed by many to be a critical ingredient in determining life success. Rather than a crude measure of skills such as writing, math and reasoning, emotional intelligence is more concerned with the ability of people to detect, perceive and act upon other peoples' emotions. Given this definition, it's easy to see why someone with a gift in this area may do very well. But is it something innate or something you can learn? The jury is still out there, but at one basic level it can be interpreted as simply being considerate to the needs of others.

At the opposite end of the spectrum is the medical condition known as *autism*. Autistic people are unable to detect emotions and feelings in others. One of the medical evaluations that determines if an individual is autistic is known as the *Sally-Anne Test*. When this is performed, an autistic person is shown two dolls, one called Sally and the other called Anne. Sally has an item, like a marble, under a basket in front of her. She leaves the scene and while she is away, Anne takes the marble out of Sally's basket and hides it. When Sally returns, the test-taker is asked where she will look for her marble. Usually children will realize that Sally will go and look for it under her own basket first, where she is expecting it to be. An autistic child will be unable to comprehend this, and will assume that Sally will go and look for it wherever Anne has hidden it.

The evidence suggests that the earlier social skills are nurtured, the better. In research from the United Kingdom, investigators followed a group of children from the ages of 3 to 12.[22] Three-year-olds were shown a series of pictures that they looked at with their mothers. Researchers looked at whether the mothers talked to their children about the mental state and emotions of the people in the pictures, or were they more concerned with other more objective things about the picture? When the children were older, other tests were administered to assess their social understanding. One of the tasks involved watching scenes from the hit television comedy, "The Office." From the age of 8, it was noticed that many of the children were beginning to feel terrible when they saw the hapless embarrassing boss in action! By the age of 12, they were found to do as well as their mothers, showing a similar level of social sophistication. But here was the difference. In the children whose mothers had previously been found to talk to them more emotionally about the pictures, testing showed a higher level of social understanding. This was *independent* of the mothers' own IQ or social understanding. The researchers concluded that mothers who talk to their children about peoples' feelings, beliefs, needs and intentions, developed better social understanding in their children than mothers who didn't do this. A big part of someone's emotional intelligence is likely to be shaped at an early age.

Be in good company

The people you surround yourself with play an important role in your life. After my first year of medical school I worked for the summer at London's Heathrow Airport, in the import administration department. It was a beautiful summer, and there was a group of students, all of a similar age, working together doing what was actually quite a mundane job sorting paper records. Looking back at all the other temporary work I had when I was still a student, and even all my jobs as a physician, that one summer job was simply the most enjoyable work I have ever done! All of us would have great interactions during the day, I met some really interesting people, and we all played sports and went out after work. Yet we still got the work done too. It was a truly amazing job that I have very happy memories of. I don't remember ever feeling stressed about needing to sort through thousands of import documents, or getting bored at work. I actually relished arriving at work. It was just because I was working with a terrific group of people and we would have a lot of fun and keep encouraging each other. Similar things also happened to me in medical school and as a doctor. I would go on rotations to the most rural, "un-happening" places—areas and hospitals that were considered dreary and depressing. But working with the right people and having an interactive team always made the job much more enjoyable. I would often end up liking and learning from some of these rotations much more so than the ones in big cities with large university hospitals. Why? Because I was surrounded by great people.

We all feel better when in good company. We can exchange stories, solicit opinions, and get feedback on our own situations. We can debate, laugh and sometimes cry together. A well-known saying goes that a problem shared is a problem halved, and it's very true. Two heads are also better than one for problem-solving. All of us have at some point faced a scenario where we've been burdened with something and feel overwhelmed, but after talking to a trusted person, feel much better. Whether it's a friend, significant other or family member, spending time with people you like and trust is very valuable. And it's always a two-way process. Just as you share your problems with another person, so must you be able to listen to theirs too. While *speaking is silver, listening is gold*.

In fact, having the right people around you can produce substantial health benefits too. In a study from Australia, researchers sought to determine whether having strong social networks with family and friends predicted longevity.[23] Almost 1,500 people over the age of 70 were studied for ten years. The results showed that those with the largest self-reported networks of friends were also likely to live the longest. Overall, the most socially active people had a staggering *22 percent higher* survival rate when compared to those with the least friends. The investigators also corrected for other factors such as baseline health, which could have confounded the results. Another large review from Brigham Young University of almost 150 smaller studies involving more than 300,000 participants from four different continents yielded an even more impressive result.[24] This time, when all the data was pooled together, there appeared to be a *50 percent increased* likelihood of survival in people with stronger social relationships. More remarkably, when this data was analyzed further, one mathematical model even suggested a *91 percent increase* in the odds of survival! These trends were consistent across males and females, different ages and initial health status.

We will talk more about happiness in the next chapter, but people with wider social circles have been found to be much more contented too. One survey from the University of Chicago showed that people with five or more close friends are *50 percent more* likely to describe themselves as "very happy" compared to those with smaller social circles.[25] The relationship with your spouse is usually the most important one in life, and research has shown that married couples are consistently happier than those who have never married.[26] Other studies have shown that people with neurotic partners are significantly less happy than those with more emotionally stable partners.[27] The advice therefore seems to be to choose wisely, because divorce is one of the most traumatic life events, and people stuck in an unhappy marriage are the unhappiest of all. The effect of having children in your life appears to be a mixed bag. Many people claim to be unhappy and stressed while they are looking after their kids, but if you ask them afterwards they say it is one of the most enjoyable and rewarding parts of their lives!

Scientists have put forward many different theories as to how having stronger relationships produces such dramatic results in terms of longevity. As well as the psychosocial mechanisms of increased social support and engagement, biological and physiological mechanisms may be activated that produce direct cardiovascular benefits. Unfortunately, however, the trend in the modern Western world is generally towards *decreased* social interactions. We are less likely to live in larger extended families, more of us live alone for longer periods of time, and we live farther away from the people we are close to. And of course, when we are talking about friends, it is paramount for us to define what a true friend is, so that we are receiving support from the right people.

Sure, friends often come and go in life, and everybody has fallings out every now and again. A sad result though of the Internet era and all its "virtual" social networks is that they tend to devalue the true meaning of a friend. Nobody can have 150 friends. Acquaintances and people you vaguely know, maybe, but *friends* no.

Thus, the clear message is to be in good company whenever you can. Never isolate yourself from those people who are important to you. Try not to lose touch with old friends and former colleagues. Send an email or call somebody each week to catch up. Meet as many new people as possible. Spend more time with family and friends at every opportunity. Have a nice dinner, an enjoyable day out, or a shopping trip—the more the better. It'll do you a world of good.

Spreading your feelings

Most of us frequently experience how quickly our emotions can affect others and how their emotions can affect us. We walk into a room full of laughter and feel like laughing ourselves. We walk into a room full of sadness and quickly feel the same sense of somberness. In an experiment from Germany a group of volunteers was shown a series of photos, and it was found that feelings of happiness and sadness were significantly evoked in the viewer after looking at the picture for just *half a second!*[28] This effect has been shown to work over the longer term too. One large study looked into this concept, calling it the *infectivity of emotions.*[29] Using data from the

Framingham Heart Study, subjects were assessed every three years and classified as either content, discontent or neutral. Complex social connection charts were constructed on the basis of family, friends, coworkers and neighbors. Any change in scores was noted between assessments, and detailed mathematical models were used to look for any potential spread of emotions. What they showed was a definite and clear *spread* of emotional states between socially connected individuals. In other words, a type of "infectious spread." In further analysis of the Framingham data, another combined team looked at information on more than 4,700 people over a twenty year period.[30] Once again, there were definite clusters of happiness, and the researchers calculated that someone who lived within a mile of a friend who became happy had his or her own probability of happiness increased by *25 percent*.

Results like this tell us that we are better off trying to surround ourselves with the happiest people, at least to increase the chances of our own happiness. Likewise, we are also capable of extending our own feelings to others. Obviously, sometimes the situation does not allow for happiness. It's not a simple case of just finding happy people to hang out with. But in general, the more we are around positive emotions, the more they will spread to us too. This is an everyday effect worth remembering.

Better daily interactions

Unfortunately in today's spinning modern world, the type of direct communication that we have all evolved to participate in is becoming less and less common. Nowadays we have telephones, emails, video conferencing and text messages. Obviously none of this is as adequate for our ability to satisfactorily interact. We need to connect personally and the only way this can happen is when we are talking face-to-face. Have you ever heard about somebody second-hand, dealt with them by telephone or email and come to a decision that you didn't like them? Have you then gone on to meet them in person and had your opinion completely shattered and thought to yourself, *Gosh, they are nowhere near as bad as I thought!* It's a common occurrence. This is particularly relevant in the work setting, and is why when you need to communicate an important message, face-to-face direct meetings are always the best option. Whenever there's a communication void at work, it always tends to be filled with rumors and hearsay. Addressing this has proven to be better for organizations' bottom lines too, as statistics show that companies that promote effective communication by addressing employee concerns and training managers in good communication skills have an almost 50 percent higher total return to shareholders over a five-year period.[31] One of the real drawbacks of bad financial times is that many organizations tend to neglect these areas. But this is actually the time when people need to be sticking together and communicating more, *not* less. Another common cutback is in the area of business travel, where it has been estimated that for every dollar invested, companies can reap an impressive $12.50 in revenue, and conversely lose up to 30 percent of business without in-person meetings.[32] That's not really surprising. Many of the new ideas that lead to great things arise from chance meetings and if you are not meeting face-to-face with your clients, these can't happen.

Interacting with people we perceive as difficult can be one of the hardest things to do. Everyone knows people whom they find tough to deal with—whether they are uncooperative, know-it-alls, fault-finding or just never satisfied. If you've tried everything, then it may be time to accept that you just don't agree, and move on. Even the most amicable people in the world can't get on with *everybody* at all times. Remember too that civility and respect is a two-way street. If you've climbed the career ladder, it's all too easy sometimes to forget what things were like when you were at the bottom. I'm always amazed by colleagues of mine whom I've seen progress, and then turn into the types of superiors that they once hated themselves! No matter how far you have gone, keep in mind how tough things can be for those still working their way up.

As human beings, we are naturally primed to be *wary of the other tribe*. People who are different from us in any way always tend to initiate a fearful reaction at first. This can work on any social level—in your neighborhood, in the mall or at work. How often, for instance, in the workplace have you heard about the "people in HR" or the "people in accounts" being one way or another? We all probably realize deep inside how silly it is to pitch one group of people against another like this and lump them all together. But the less we regularly meet them, the more these types of scenario keep playing out. Some companies are even getting around this by mixing workspaces to promote familiarity among people in different departments. That's a great idea. Whatever situation we are in, be it the new neighbor who doesn't fit into the mold or the worker in the different department, when we meet them face-to-face we usually realize that what President Clinton said in his speech is true. We are almost all the same, and we all want the same basic things in life.

Human contact is, and always will be, a primitive and basic need. It will be desired even if one day we are living in space! Social interactions enable bonding, support, inspiration, and an opportunity for other interchanges such as humor. As you've seen from the research, how we connect with other people forms a vital part of our well-being, and also has a direct impact on our health. Much of our lives are defined by our interactions with others, and whether we like it or not we are involved in these all the time, both with new people and those we already know, from those very first instantaneous judgments to the emotional flow that occurs with our loved ones. It can sometimes appear that some people are born to be better communicators than others. But like everything else in life, things can always be enhanced with practice. Whatever you do to improve these interactions, from allowing yourself more time to judge, making more eye contact, smiling, complimenting or being more amicable and considerate, the benefits are there to be gained. Simple virtues are also always the right ones. Things like openness, transparency, sincerity, honesty and empathy. Using them in your daily life will rarely fail you. Making the most out of your daily interactions is not only in your best interests, but also in others' as well. Better relationships will bring you more success and substantially boost your physical and emotional health.

HIGH PERCENTAGE SOCIAL WELLNESS STEPS

- Avoid instantaneous judgments about people

    Don't always trust those first instincts, but at the same time make a good first impression

- Look people in the eye

    Communicating face-to-face is what we are wired to do

- Smile more

    Be in situations that keep you smiling

- Compliment

    Pay one whenever one is due

- Apologize

    Say sorry if you're at fault

- Adopt high-power poses

    Base your postures on maximal expansiveness

- Get along with those around you

    Be flexible, it can help you go far

- Keep good company

    Surround yourself with family and friends at every opportunity

- Be in happy company

    To encourage healthy emotional flow

CHAPTER SEVEN

LIFE WELLNESS: THE PURSUIT OF HAPPINESS

In the late 18th century a group of inspired men led a young new country to freedom from a mighty empire. When the founding fathers proclaimed the Declaration of Independence on July 4, 1776, they also brought forth a new idea never before seen in any national manifesto. As well as the inalienable rights including life and liberty, the citizens also had a right to the *pursuit of happiness*. This was a revolutionary idea, although it now seems intrinsic to life itself. The pursuit of happiness is what everyone wants. On a purely psychosocial level, the terms happiness and well-being are interchangeable. Can we really have one without the other?

Hundreds of thousands of years ago, our ancestors took the decision to diverge from the rest of the animal kingdom and step out of the cave to explore pastures new. We built villages and formed little societies. We developed tools and unique methods of transport. We built even bigger buildings that eventually formed cities. We crossed land and then made vessels to navigate the seas. In the last century we took to the skies and then even left the planet. Of course there is a dark side too, with terrible fighting, disputes and wars being just as much part of our collective history. The limitless scope of our potential is almost matched by our capacity for destruction. But on the brighter side, we are all primed to aspire and reach higher in pursuit of better things.

The word *success* is a universally positive word. Have you ever met anybody who tells you that they don't want to be successful? It's just as unlikely as somebody not wanting to be healthy! There are very few words with such a glowing undertone that are met with such universal approval. Success, after all, can apply to so many different areas of life, be they family, educational, career or financial. Everyone wants (and needs) to feel successful according to his or her own personal goals. Having these aims and goals to strive for is almost as important a part of our lives as eating and sleeping. Even if you eat the best diet possible and exercise like an elite athlete, if you don't have life goals then you are unlikely to feel a true sense of well-being or happiness. From relatively minor accomplishments such as completing the front room decor, to a long-term endeavor like pursuing an educational qualification, achieving successes—both small and large—is what drives us each and every day. Experiencing the personal joy from reaching our goals can be one of the most satisfying experiences in life, especially if we have worked hard in doing so.

Conventional wisdom and assumption would suggest that success leads to happiness. When we get that pay raise, we can be happy. When we buy that suburban home with a swimming pool, we will be happy. When our kids finish college, then we will be happy. It's a common mindset. We need to achieve our goals in order to be happy, right? In recent years, however, this traditional relationship between success and happiness has well and truly been turned on its head, because research is now showing that it's frequently actually the other way round. Namely, that happiness *leads* to success.[1] Happy people are more likely to engage in behaviors that are conducive to positive outcomes. The lens through which we view the world and react to challenges has a direct bearing on what we get out of it.

What's motivating you?

Motivation is the initial driving force behind all of our endeavors. It can be the result of many different thought processes. Among other things, we can be motivated by prestige, title, money, self-fulfillment or even pleasing others. These forces become more pertinent when we are working towards long-term goals. For example, you can be driven to pursue an extra qualification for your own betterment, for the knowledge itself, for that job promotion or for that increased paycheck! Lately, psychologists have been increasingly studying the fundamentals of our motivations, and what determines successful versus unsuccessful subsequent actions. To achieve a life goal, we obviously need to remain focused and dedicated, often over long time periods. The question is, what characteristic thought patterns lead people to be better at achieving their objectives? The results are surprising and interesting, because it's not necessarily all about having a carrot dangled in front of us.

The world of psychology has classified motivation as either being *intrinsic* or *extrinsic*. You may remember that we touched upon something similar for weight management. Broadly speaking, *intrinsic motivation* is the drive to achieve a goal because of your own desire for self-improvement and personal growth. *Extrinsic motivation* is the ambition to succeed for other, more external reasons, like power, money or fame. You may ask, what difference does it make as long as we achieve what we are aiming for? The reason it matters is because whichever camp your motivation falls into has profound implications on your likelihood of success, and also of satisfaction. Research has consistently shown that intrinsically motivated people fare better in their endeavors than those who are extrinsically motivated. Doing something for purely external rewards will not only be less fulfilling, but can also significantly reduce performance levels and the quality of your work. This effect is especially true when your task needs you to be creative.

In one cleverly designed experiment from Boston, researchers investigated this phenomenon on a small task level.[2] They took 72 young adult volunteer writers and asked them to write two brief poems consisting of five lines each. But there was a catch. After writing the first poem, the volunteers were divided into three separate groups. The first group completed a questionnaire that made them focus on their intrinsic reasons for writing, asking them to rank the importance of seven reasons for writing, such as enjoying self-expression, achieving new insights and playing with words. The second group filled out a different questionnaire, focusing on purely extrinsic reasons such as impressing others and getting financial rewards. The third group acted as a control group, and was given no reasons for writing. Everyone was then asked to write the second five-line poem. When all of the poems were assessed and rated by an independent panel of twelve judges, they found that there were no differences in creativity of the first poems written. There was, however, a very *big* difference with the second poems. The group that was primed to focus on extrinsic reasons for writing was judged by the independent panel to be significantly *less* creative and produced lower-quality poems than the other two groups. In other words, just getting these talented writers to think about external motivations for a few brief minutes caused them to waver in their talents, and produce a lower quality of writing immediately afterwards. The writers had been led astray by external thinking!

Other experiments have shown that our interest in a task can actually decline with extrinsic rewards. One study of schoolchildren who initially had a high interest in drawing with a marker found that when they began to compete for an award, their level of interest significantly decreased and they produced lower-quality drawings when compared to a group of schoolchildren who were not competing for an award.[3]

The evidence also points to intrinsically motivated people faring better in terms of psychological health. In an intriguing study, psychologists sought to find out what led a group of college graduates to purse their goals immediately after leaving college and what effect this may have on their physical health.[4] This group was especially good to study, because the post-college period is the time when most young adults are left to their own devices for the first time, and are no longer in an institutionalized, regimented system. The researchers used psychological questionnaires to determine the baseline aspirations of almost 250 graduates, most of whom then responded to a follow-up assessment one and two years later. The questions were based on an index that measured life satisfaction, self-esteem and physical symptoms. The results showed that when people attained intrinsic aspirations related to personal growth, relationships and community, this was more likely to be associated with positive psychological health. On the contrary, attainment of extrinsic aspirations such as wealth, fame and image, was found to be related to indicators of ill-being.

On the surface, such studies confirm what we already know and see on a day-to-day basis. People who are focused on extrinsic reasons for wanting to do something always fare worse than people who are intrinsically motivated. This latter group not only has more success, but also gets more enjoyment and satisfaction from their endeavors. That's not to diminish or devalue the importance of some extrinsic values too. It's great to get the position, the title and the financial rewards. Realistically, these factors are a potent driving force in life, but they should never be the *sole* focus of your pursuits.

Being driven purely for these reasons will never bring you the best benefits. When it comes to motivation, therefore, it's not enough to have the skills or understanding to succeed. In order for your achievement to be optimal, the reasons for your motivation have to be right. In our everyday lives, this doesn't necessarily mean changing goals, but can simply involve reframing them. Let's take a common real-life example—wanting a promotion. You will reap greater rewards if you see this as an opportunity for learning new things and making more of a difference. If you just view a promotion as simply a way to make more money or have a more impressive title (all of which may be true) then you will not get the full well-being boost that comes with real accomplishment. In fact, the most accomplished people often say they would do their job for free!

So whenever you are working towards an important life goal, ask yourself what the true reasons are for wanting to achieve the goal, and make sure it has more to do with internal, rather than external, reasons. No advice could be better than trying to *find a cause bigger than yourself*. You will be more likely to be successful, fulfilled and happier too.

Avoid procrastination and start broadcasting your plans

Procrastination is a problem for most of us at different times. We are constantly putting things off for another day. The problem is that all too often, that tomorrow never comes. One Canadian research study on procrastination yielded some interesting findings (and rumor has it the study was published later than expected).[5] A large proportion of people define themselves as chronic procrastinators, and these figures seem to be going up. This is partly because we have so many more distractions nowadays. Procrastinators generally have less confidence in themselves and, contrary to popular belief, perfectionists seem to fare better in achieving their goals because they worry more about putting things off. The author of the article even devised a mathematical equation to predict procrastination! Everyday procrastination may not have any consequences at first, but when we are talking about something important like retirement planning, it soon becomes a major problem.

Remember, *Rome wasn't built in a day*. It takes time, focus and energy to achieve any long-term goal. Suppose you've thought about moving and have known for a while that it's what you really want to do. Your family situation is flexible and there are no major obstacles in your way. What are you waiting for? You can start doing the serious research right away. Work out how much the property is where you want to move. Inquire tentatively about whatever it is that matters to you most, whether it's the job situation, schools or the community environment. If you start with these small steps, you may be surprised at how quickly a wave can carry you forward. But the point is that you have to start the serious movement. The naysayers will likely be everywhere, telling you not to take that risk. But if you truly have that itch to try something new, then what's the worst that could happen? Move back? The same goes for anything else. You are thinking of a career change and are miserable in your current job. Then you don't need to stay miserable. You can start writing that resume or working on that extra qualification now. Even if you know it's something that you can't do yet, just starting the process is a great first step. Basically, you're doing a little bit whenever you can to work your way towards your dream. The famous 19th century British novelist Anthony Trollope wisely observed that *a small daily task, if it be really daily, will beat the labours of a spasmodic Hercules.*

When you do have that plan or endeavor in mind, don't be shy about telling friends and family about it, because it may also increase your chances of success. In one study, almost 150 adults from a variety of different backgrounds were assigned to five different groups according to how they dealt with achieving goals.[6] These included primarily work-related goals, such as getting organized, increasing productivity or completing a project. The first group had an unwritten goal and the second had a written goal. The third group had a written goal with action commitments and the fourth group also had to tell a friend about their commitments. The fifth group did the same as the fourth group, but also gave regular weekly progress reports to their friend. After four weeks, all the participants were asked to rate their progress and degree to which they accomplished their goals. The results were quite telling. The fifth group achieved significantly *more* than all other groups. The other achievement rates were roughly in order of group number. In other words, the more commitments you show, either in writing or by telling people, the better your chances for success. This makes sense. Few people are happy reporting no progress when they are asked about their endeavors, and having a certain amount of pressure can be a good thing. This could work equally well for family or friends. And you don't necessarily have to annoy all your friends by sending them weekly progress reports! Just telling and advertising your plans a bit and feeling accountable may be enough to push you even further to succeed. With written goals too, remember what we learned earlier about weight loss charts helping to motivate you? It's the same principle in action here. Use a simple visual to guide you in your progress. That's why many "battlerooms" of organizations will have whiteboards displaying their progress to their leading executives. It's just about visually charting out their aims and path to success.

Money

My mom is full of great anecdotes and observations, and once told me that anything *natural* gives us a warning when we have had enough of it. We eat too much, drink too much, run too much or are exposed to the weather for an excessive time, and our bodies will send us a warning signal that we shouldn't go any further. Unfortunately, this doesn't apply to *unnatural* things—like money. We are never able to get enough of all the unnatural things we have in our lives.

We may as well just admit it. Money is one of the main factors our modern day lives revolve around, and no discussion on well-being would be complete without mentioning it. We need money to buy food, warmth and just about everything else. Without it, there's no way we can feel secure. We are prone to measuring our own worth according to how much we make, and kids will make life career decisions based upon how much they are going to earn. So we've already seen that it may not be the best sole motivator, but is it truly the root of all evils that some people make it out to be? And if most of us are really chasing after it, will it bring us happiness when we acquire it? It's a question as old as time itself. Does being rich and owning possessions make you satisfied? The intuitive answer has to be *no*. Consider this. Over the last several decades we all have much more money than ever before. Most people have life luxuries that would have been unthinkable for their parents to own. Our personal income has increased by more than two-and-a-half times over the last 50 years, yet no consistent evidence has shown any corresponding increase in our happiness levels. We also know from our own carefree times in university or college when most of us had little money, that we may even have been happier than we were afterwards *with* more money!

Yet at the same time, it's not that simple either. All of us would similarly agree that we'd much rather be rich and happy than poor and happy. Conversely, it's obviously better to be rich and unhappy than poor and unhappy! All else being equal, having money always seems to be better. So what exactly does the scientific evidence tell us about how money correlates with our life satisfaction?

One massive survey of almost 450,000 Americans looked into this precise question. The results found that money can indeed buy happiness, but only up to about $75,000 a year.[7] This may surprise a lot of people. Although it may still be above many peoples' household income (the median US household number hovers above $50,000), it isn't exactly millionaire territory either. The researchers found that, in general, emotional well-being didn't change beyond this level, even though people could *feel* more successful with increasing income. Someone who moved from $100,000 to $200,000, for instance, was not found to be happier on a day-to-day basis. This backs up the widely held theory that having money increases happiness when it lifts people solidly into the middle class, but little beyond that. Once you feel relatively comfortable, more doesn't necessarily improve things. Of course, for many people, the problem is getting into that middle class in the first place. Nevertheless, all those dreams about how happy and fulfilling your life would be if you were a millionaire aren't necessarily well-founded. The most important thing is feeling secure and not worried about where your next meal or mortgage payment is coming from.

What defines *comfort* is also determined by those around you and to whom you are comparing yourself. Comfortable in suburban America is very different from comfortable in a remote jungle tribe. Humans, being the competitive animals that we are, are prone to measuring ourselves according to what other people have. Which brings us to the next major theory with regards to money and happiness—namely, that it's not how much *you* have that matters, but how much money your *neighbor* has. The term neighbor here has biblical connotations, because it can be whichever person you are thinking about. Psychologists in the United Kingdom looked at the results of a survey of more than 85,000 people and found that although a person's salary is important, their social standing actually matters more to their happiness.[8] Earning 2 million pounds a year will not make you happy if all your family and friends make 3 million a year. This is a very human trait, and is why absolute income is so arbitrary when it comes to measures of happiness. We have to *feel* ahead. Two further concepts that underlie this are the *reference income* hypothesis and the *rank income* hypothesis. The reference income hypothesis argues that people compare their wealth to the normal, or average, of a comparison group and subsequently derive life satisfaction. The rank income hypothesis, on the other hand, suggests that people only care about what position their income ranks among those around them. So it's nothing to do with the average, but only your own individual rank among your peers. Unsurprisingly, the latter theory has been gaining increased traction of late. This may also be the reason too that communism never worked! People tend to gain more satisfaction if they know they are ahead of others, and also lend more weight to upward comparisons than downward ones. For example, we will be more inclined to focus on the few people earning more than we do, rather than the many who earn less. And bearing in mind what we said before about rising incomes for the last several decades not affecting happiness levels, these theories make perfect sense. When thinking about money, it's usually how much our neighbor is making that we become fixated upon. Most people would rather earn $50,000 a year if everyone important to them earned $25,000, than make $75,000 a year in a group that is making $100,000!

If you find it difficult to believe that there are any unhappy millionaires, just read some of the numerous news articles about lottery winners whose lives turned completely sour after their win, and who years later are left wishing that they had never won. This may seem incomprehensible, but the dozens of stories are right there in front of us. It's because *how* we acquire the money also decides if we are satisfied with it or not. Lottery winners will usually quickly return back to their baseline contentment once all the initial excitement fades away. On the contrary, people will maintain far more satisfaction when they have earned their cash themselves, as opposed to just being given it. This effect is actually based on our brain science, and was highlighted in an experiment from Emory University.[9] A group of 16 volunteers was asked to either play a challenging computer game for money, or was given a sealed envelope containing the money without earning it on the game. The volunteers also underwent MRI scans of their brains. After looking at the scans, the researchers found that the reward centers of the brain were activated whenever a volunteer received money. However, a region of the brain called the *striatum* was stimulated only when the volunteers had to work for their reward. This was an important discovery because the striatum is associated with feelings of pleasure. Playing a challenging game and subsequently being rewarded appeared to activate more pleasure centers than just being given the money without working for it. We can see this real-life effect in many people who suddenly get given a lot of money out of the blue, whether from a lottery or from a trust fund. They are never as satisfied as they would have been had they actually *earned* the money themselves. We are just not built to get significant rewards without working for them.

When we do have the money, what we spend it on is also crucial for determining how much pleasure we derive from it. The evidence consistently shows that people gain much more happiness from spending money on life experiences rather than on material possessions. In one study, participants were asked to answer questions about their recent purchases and how they felt about them.[10] The results revealed that people who bought experiences such as a trip to the theater experienced greater happiness levels than people who made material purchases. Another survey of 12,000 people conducted on behalf of a large financial institution found that when faced with a choice, the majority of people said that choosing an experiential purchase over a material one made them more content.[11] Most of us can probably relate to these findings. First, we don't get bored of happy memories the same way we do with a material object. Good memories can bloom over time and don't get old like your new shoes. It's also more fun to talk about a great trip than it is your new material purchase (one would hope). The two don't necessarily need to always be separate either—there can be overlap between material goods and experiences, such as that new mountain bike or special event outfit. But the overall message is clear. Money spent on experiences is more likely to make you happy than money spent on material goods. Chasing after material possessions all the time is a sure-fire happiness killer and a no-win game. After you buy that nice car, you will soon want another one, and then another, even better one. We tend to overestimate how much pleasure we are likely to derive from possessing more, and the thrill of a material purchase quickly vanishes. So if you really want money, let it be for all the great vacations you can go on rather than all the new possessions you can buy. This doesn't mean you need to live like a monk and not enjoy material luxuries, but it's something to keep in mind. Let's take a hypothetical scenario. Imagine you arrive home one day and your house is burning down. You only have time to grab a few items. What will you get? Well, assuming that nobody is in there (when it may be a good idea to grab them first) most people would probably go for the photo albums or home videos. I know I would. These are the irreplaceable items. All the other expensive material goods that you worked so hard to purchase, like the flat-screen television and leather sofa, are totally replaceable.

Finally, none of this suggests that you shouldn't try to make money. If you want to make money, then more power to you, but making it your sole aim will not make you particularly happy or fulfilled (remember the motivation studies), and even if you become rich, the evidence doesn't bode well for hugely increased happiness either. Look at the people around you. Are the richest people you know also the happiest people? Unlikely. The most valuable assets are the things that cannot be bought. Things like family, friends, health, knowledge and time. Perhaps we would do well to remember the tale of Alexander the Great, who conquered everywhere he went and created one of the largest empires in ancient history. Legend has it that before dying he gave detailed instructions for his funeral procession. One of his requests was that his hands be left open, dangling outwards for all the world to see that in spite of his vast possessions and unlimited wealth, *there goes Alexander the Great leaving empty-handed.*

Optimism: The amazing power of positivity

Okay, some people simply always appear be more optimistic and positive, and others more cynical and negative. Is the glass half-empty or half-full? Are you an *optimist* or a *pessimist*? Perhaps people are simply wired one way or another. Or maybe we become a certain way given our own personal experiences. There's no doubt that many people have suffered terrible experiences in life that have made them prone to having a more negative outlook. Going against this are the people who despite their adversities still maintain positivity. Then there's the curious group who appear to have a lot going for them, but just appear to see nothing but obstacles!

A relatively new concept that has been flourishing in recent years is based on something called *positive psychology*. This movement has evolved in response to the negative psychology that had dominated scientific research for decades. In the mid-1990s, it was estimated that scientific journals published about 100 studies on sadness for every one study on happiness. Sad (again, no pun intended) but true. So instead of focusing on the psychology that underlies positive and successful outcomes, the science was only concentrating on the negativity and failure that underpinned bad outcomes. Your mom probably already told you many times when you were little to stay positive and hopeful (especially around exam times) but this may have been more than just motherly advice. The power of positive thinking is now being proven again and again, and research is showing why this approach is actually much better for us too.

Let's start first with some simple definitions. Optimism is defined by a series of traits including determination, resilience and yes, happiness. A big determinant of someone's level of optimism is what psychologists call their unique *explanatory style*. In a nutshell, this is how someone explains whatever obstacles and setbacks are encountered, and can be divided according to three criteria. It can be *unstable* or *stable*, *specific* or *global*, and *external* or *internal*. Perplexing? Take an example. If somebody suffers a negative life event, say a job rejection, an explanation of why this happened will either be: "These rejections will keep coming (stable), this is going to affect everything I do now (global), and it's all because of me (internal)." On the other hand, someone else's reaction might be: "This is just a one-time rejection (unstable), this is only a temporary thing (specific), and it's not my fault (external)." Can you see the very different ways of interpreting the same event and how they relate to pessimism and optimism? As far as explanatory style goes, an unstable, specific and external reasoning is a marker for optimism.

This is obviously the difference between someone who gives up easily and someone who keeps on trying. The more negative approach, at its worst, can also lead to a state of mind known as *learned helplessness*, which is the opposite of taking charge of a situation. This occurs when someone believes that he or she has no control over a desired objective and that any repeated attempts to succeed are futile.

In all areas of life, optimists are able to pick themselves up more quickly and shrug off a brief setback. Traditionally it was always thought that ability and motivation were the only markers of success, but now many psychologists have added this third factor of positivity and optimism. We've already read in the stress section how dwelling on things can bring you down. Positivity involves the least possible dwelling time and a quick turnaround time to moving on to the next step.

Businesses have known for a long time that optimists, especially in sales and marketing careers, always do better and outperform their more pessimistic colleagues, by as much as 40 percent.[12] This can actually be extended to almost any other career, and we all probably know a lot of real-life examples. New tools are even being devised to assess peoples' baseline positivity before they are hired, not so much to weed out the negative ones, but just as much to make sure that they are going to be placed in the right jobs. Even if an individual is more inclined towards being a pessimist, some companies offer training courses to help them not feel dejected too quickly. Let's take somebody working in sales to attract new clients to the company, a job that by nature has a high failure rate. An optimist will take rejection after rejection and just move on, with confidence and a real belief that he or she will eventually succeed. A pessimist will get perhaps two rejections in a row and feel downbeat, wrongly taking it as a personal rejection. A great friend of mine, who I grew up with, was never very successful academically when he was young but was always good at talking to people, had a gift for persuasion, and is a remarkable optimist. He's a sincere guy who just loves to talk! He is also very resilient and good at taking a rejection on the cheek—something, to be fair, most of us are not. After finishing his university studies, he got what seemed like a mediocre job in the sales department of a large software company. He quickly excelled, and gained promotion after promotion. His clients love him and he is now traveling the world securing multimillion-dollar contracts. Admittedly, his success is not because of any great technical skills or know-how. He is just born to talk to clients and engage them in a strategy to improve their business. His industry can be volatile, and clients come and go. He once told me that he sees other people in his company feel down or get depressed after a negative setback, such as a client being overly demanding or taking their business to another company, and feels despair himself! He said that these colleagues moan and feel rejected for hours and days, while he just picks up the phone and *moves on*, either working out a solution or focusing on the next client. For him, resilience and optimism are natural.

Let's say you have invested in shares that suddenly go up and make you a lot of money. A pessimist will see this as a stroke of luck while an optimist will see this as a clever investment. You fall and hurt your leg slightly. A pessimist will be cursing his or her luck and going over and over the events. An optimist will thank God for being alive and the fact that it was only a minor injury! The choice in viewing the world through a glass half empty or half full is totally yours.

So in what other areas of life has optimism proven to be the best way forward? Let's start with academics. In research from Australia, a clear link was found between optimism and problem-solving capacity.[13] Those with belief were clearly more likely to succeed. Students did better when they believed that not knowing was *temporary* and could be overcome through their own personal effort. In fact, the concept of *academic optimism* is all the more attractive because it emphasizes the potential of schools to overcome the power of socioeconomic factors and be in charge of their own fate. Another study from the same institution on Grades 5 and 6 schoolchildren who were taped by video camera, and then viewed by experts, found that richer learning occurred when all students were optimistic.[14]

On the other end of the age spectrum, one team of researchers showed that having more positivity and optimism could actually lower the risk of falling.[15] Their study followed 500 older people for one year, and divided them according to personality traits. The results revealed that anxious, negative people who had a low fall risk, but high perceived risk, would actually fall *more*. On the other hand, the positive "stoic" people who had a high actual risk but low perceived risk, would fall *less*. The conclusion was that a positive life outlook with more optimism and confidence appeared to be protective against falling.

In the last chapter you read about the dramatic effects that a smile can have, and obviously, smiling is also a general marker for positivity. In a series of studies, similar effects have been discovered for trait optimism. In one of the most famous, researchers conducted an experiment involving 180 Catholic nuns from Baltimore and Milwaukee.[16] Back in 1930, each nun had written a brief autobiography, at an average age of just 22. These autobiographies were analyzed and classified according to writing style, using a scoring system to determine a more positive emotional content versus a more negative one. When they then looked at what subsequently happened to the nuns, they found a strong relationship between the writing style in the autobiographies and their survival rates at ages 75 to 95. Overall, the nuns who wrote autobiographies with the most positive emotional content had a *two and a half times* higher survival rate compared to those with the least positivity. This was even more remarkable given the fact that the autobiographies were written almost six decades before!

This result was no fluke. Another study from Duke University looked at more than 7,000 students who completed a scientific personality questionnaire in the mid-1960s, and traced these people more than 40 years later.[17] The analysis showed that the most optimistic individuals, as measured by the scale, had a *42 percent increased* longevity compared with the most pessimistic. Perhaps unsurprisingly, heart disease risk in particular appears to be made worse by a more pessimistic outlook. In a paper aptly titled "Is the Glass Half Empty or Half Full?," investigators from Harvard studied this effect on 1,300 relatively healthy men who lived in the Boston area.[18] Using the same personality questionnaire, these men were studied for a decade. This time, the results were even more impressive, with men who had high levels of optimism having a *56 percent reduced* risk of heart attacks and cardiovascular mortality compared to the most pessimistic. These patterns held true even after correcting for alcohol intake and smoking. Indeed, this cardiovascular protective phenomenon has been proven equally in women too. Using data from almost 100,000 women from the Women's Health Initiative Study over an eight-year follow-up, optimists were found to have a *30 percent reduced* rate of cardiovascular mortality compared to the most pessimistic.[19] The study also found that women classed as being the most "cynical and hostile" had a *16 percent higher* total mortality and a *23 percent higher* cancer related mortality.

And so the terrific effects of positivity keep going on and on. One more study of 670 men even found that optimists had significantly higher levels of lung capacity and a slower rate of decline in lung function over time![20] In fact, it's probable that if almost any disease or condition was studied, the likelihood of an improvement with optimism is highly likely. The funny thing is that most doctors observe these effects on a daily basis anyway. People who are positive and optimistic always appear to do better, frequently recovering much faster from their illness than their pessimistic counterparts. I see this with every condition under the sun, from heart, lung, kidney, liver, brain and musculoskeletal ailments. People with belief and a sunny outlook always seem to bounce back quicker. While this may be partly mediated through peoples' own perception of their condition, my own experience has convinced me that something else is at work too. Patients often ask me when they are lying sick in their hospital bed if they should be doing anything else to aid their immediate recovery. I always tell them to just stay as optimistic as possible! This may be easy for me to say, but realistically, what other choice do we have? As you have read, these fascinating studies point in only one direction. *Optimism is good for your health.* They also pose a deeper question that has been asked for thousands of years, but may never be entirely answered. Where does the link between mind and body begin, and where does it end? The precise reasons for these dramatic improvements and high percentages are as yet still debated by scientists. It's conceivable that on a biological level, being optimistic produces physiological and biochemical changes similar to a de-stressing effect. This could then be manifested through improved cardiovascular parameters. Nobody knows for sure yet. Nevertheless, the statistical benefits that you've just read about are of a magnitude that pharmaceutical companies can only dream of.

It's certainly true that a large part of our explanatory style is ingrained into our personality. Life experiences also play a significant role in shaping our attitudes. Who knows what setbacks may have occurred in those Catholic nuns' early lives to make them a little bit more pessimistic in their outlook? It's not just a case of clicking your fingers and suddenly having a more positive frame of mind. Changes take time. But as we've learned from the concept of neural plasticity, our brain is capable of rebuilding itself and remodeling according to our experiences, and just as negative events can produce harmful changes, so can positive thinking bring about the benefits. In this way, our levels of optimism are not set, but can be trained. In an experiment involving 120 freshmen who were at risk for depression based on their pessimistic explanatory style, researchers randomly assigned them to either an 8-week cognitive behavioral treatment in the form of weekly 2-hour optimism seminars with homework assignments, or to a control group.[21] When the freshmen were assessed 6 to 30 months later, it was found that the seminar group had better physical health than the controls, with fewer reported symptoms and doctor visits. Learning some positivity skills produced clear benefits. It wasn't totally set at all.

Now does any of this mean that optimists don't suffer failure or illness? Of course not. But the results are pretty clear. Optimistic traits are more likely to bring you global benefits, for your health, well-being and life success. Positive people have more self-belief and are willing to take risks that later pay off. They believe that they are masters of their own fate, with fewer factors out of their control. Remember, expectations of success or failure are frequently *self-fulfilling prophecies*. Belief that one will succeed often produces overachievement, and the belief that one will fail produces underachievement. Even research in sports has shown that teams with a more collective optimistic explanatory style perform better than pessimistic ones.[22] Positive people are more likely to have stronger social support networks and always tend to be more relaxed and less depressive. They are certainly more likely to smile and we already know what that does! Pessimists will tend to magnify small situations and discount the many positives, overly focusing on the one bad thing. So if you think you may be a pessimist, ask yourself whether your beliefs are irrational and self-defeating. Replace those bad thoughts with more positive ones whenever you can.

It's important to realize too that optimism doesn't involve being blind to what's ahead of you and negating the true nature of any mountain you may have to climb. Blind optimism that ignores all the risks and dangers is foolish. Pessimism isn't necessarily entirely bad either, and can also serve a purpose at times. Imagine for a moment a treasury secretary or military commander who was totally optimistic and took massive risks all the time. That wouldn't be good. Pessimism becomes bad when it hinders you or makes you engage excessively in self-blame.

Over the years, I've heard many people debate the merits of optimism versus pessimism. There are some who even claim that pessimists fare better. Fair enough. But when push comes to shove, which one do most of us know intuitively is always the best approach? Given the choice, would anyone want to be around a pessimist rather than an optimist? The answer is obvious. Optimism is almost always the best way to go. Ultimately, it's about the belief that your life is in your own hands, and that your own endeavors and determination can change things for the better. Tomorrow will be better than today. Optimism is indeed a very *American* thing to have.

Overcoming adversity

Life is not about avoiding the storm, but about learning to dance in the rain. The ability to rise above adversity and succeed is a great trait to have, and is clearly also linked to an optimistic outlook. We can draw inspiration from those who are able to do this. People who never seem to give up in the face of impossible odds. There's the story of Robert the Bruce, King of Scots in the 14th century, one of the greatest Scottish heroes of all time. He had suffered six devastating major defeats to the English army when he decided to withdraw himself, ready to give up completely. He went into hiding in a cave, feeling depressed and downhearted. One day a spider caught his eye that was trying to weave a web. The spider was unsuccessful in its painstaking attempts over and over again, but stubbornly kept on trying to weave the web. It kept on failing, but then kept getting up again. It had tried six times when Robert the Bruce continued watching intently to see what would happen next. Then on the seventh attempt, the spider succeeded in its endeavor and successfully finished the web. Inspired by the spider's persistence, Robert the Bruce decided to keep on fighting and raised his army once more. He went on to win his next major battles, becoming one of the greatest Scottish kings of all time. Of course, there is no way to know whether this story is true, but we can all take home an important learning point. If there's something you want to do, never give up.

Research has shown that having a little adversity isn't necessarily a bad thing for your health. A combined study from New York and California investigated this question in a group of people with chronic back pain, one of the most common reasons for physician visits.[23] Almost 400 people completed a survey that asked specifically about adverse life events. Their results showed that those with some lifetime adversity reported less physical impairment, disability, and spent less time in doctors' offices, when compared to those who had experienced either no adversity or a high level of adversity. The researchers postulated that *resilience* had developed in the sufferers. They had basically become more resilient as a result of their experiences, and were not as sensitive to the pain. The authors also emphasized the word *some* prior life adversities, not a large amount, which is obviously not very desirable!

This finding shouldn't really amaze anybody. We can see from just looking around us that people who have been through a lot are often tougher. *What doesn't kill you makes you stronger.* Some people have a remarkable ability to turn apparent problems to their own advantage. From people who use the time after being laid off to pursue educational opportunities, to those with the intuition to buy stocks and shares when there's a recession, there are often many opportunities in every setback. Sometimes there is no other option than to try to make something good out of things. Let's take a simple everyday example. You are angry and finding it difficult to budget as you see gas prices rising steadily. Why not buy some shares in the petroleum company so that you are making some money too! That way, all is not lost and you are making something out of a bad situation.

There isn't anybody who hasn't encountered setbacks. Ironically, the most successful people are usually the ones who have taken the most and biggest rejections. One of my favorite phrases is actually from biblical times, about *the stone that the builders rejected becoming the cornerstone*. It happens time and time again in life and there are thousands of role models in society that we can all look up to. People who have come from relative obscurity to achieve great things, displaying magnificent persistence and self-belief. The sensational author J.K. Rowling was a single mom struggling to make ends meet before Harry Potter became famous. Barack Obama got turned away from the Democratic Convention in 2000 because he couldn't get a floor pass. Eight years later, he became President. The inspiration is all around us.

Achieving lasting happiness

It is now widely accepted that genetics accounts for only around 50 percent of our baseline level of happiness. We know from neural plasticity that we can always change our outlook on life if we try hard enough to cultivate the right parts of the brain. One large survey from Germany interviewed more than 60,000 people over a 25-year period.[24] The results showed that happiness levels were *not* pre-set, and that lifestyle choices, relationships and working life all had a significant impact. Peoples' happiness levels and life satisfaction consistently fluctuated during the study. Unsurprisingly, the study found that those who valued altruistic and family goals were much more satisfied with life. With regards to work, people who worked much more *or* much less than they wanted were unhappy. This is interesting because it shows that workaholics are not necessarily unhappy as long as they like their work! People who reported church attendance were also happier than non-religious people, proving the value of an enduring value system and moral code.

Many studies have looked into happiness levels in different countries around the world. These surveys regularly find that the most developed and richest nations don't always come out on top, which by now shouldn't be a total shock to us either. Things that make people happy vary according to where you are. For example, one survey found that happiness in the United States was most associated with personal success, while in Japan, like in many Eastern cultures, fulfilling expectations of family was more essential.[25]

Everyone is born with amazing potential and unique talents that they can offer to the world. One person might have tremendous math skills, another may have terrific people skills, and yet another may have great hand skills. We are all different, and are likely to be happiest when we take advantage of our own strengths, while also working hard to improve on our weaknesses. It's important to *play your home game* as much as possible. If, for instance, you enjoy interacting with people and meeting face-to-face, then sitting in an office working at a computer screen or number-crunching all day is unlikely to ever quite cut it for you. The type of work we do is paramount in bringing about life satisfaction. Those who are unhappy at home can sometimes still be happy at work, but the reverse is seldom seen. If you don't like your job, then there will be an inevitable carry-over to your home life too. This exists for a couple of reasons. First, remember what we said about humans being addicted to challenges. For a lot of us, these come during our work life. Second, it is the main outlet where we can actively *choose* to utilize whatever skills we have trained in. One large survey, conducted on behalf of a large bank, showed that small business owners appeared to be among the happiest of all groups.[26] The survey was conducted during a tough economic time, which makes the result even more interesting. Almost 70 percent of American small business owners described themselves as "very happy," with about 60 percent saying they are happier than the people they know. Nine out of ten of them were happier running their own business as compared to working for someone else, even though they ended up working much longer hours. Reasons included a sense of pride and accomplishment, and strong personal connections to their employees. They also liked being their own boss and being in control of decisions. While owning your own business isn't for everyone, and can undoubtedly be very stressful, it is the type of work that is most likely to unleash creativity and a sense of purpose. You are in charge and it's better than being a slave to somebody else.

Having said that, a large number small enterprises fail and don't even make enough money to sustain themselves, so it's not always the magic answer. Still, results like these delve into our psyche. We like being in *control* as much as possible. The more you can be in control, the better for your own contentment. Even if you are in an organization working for other people and don't particularly want to leave, is there anything you can do that will put you into a more powerful position? A position where you can have more charge of your own schedule and day? It will likely bring you more satisfaction.

There are many everyday practices that can help foster happiness. Simple, decent things like helping others. In one famous experiment, a group of students was asked to perform five random acts of kindness every week for six weeks.[27] These included gestures like helping out a friend, donating blood or even dropping coins into a stranger's parking meter. A separate control group was not asked to do anything. When the researchers analyzed the students' subjective feelings, their results conclusively showed that those who were performing kind acts experienced an *increase* in happiness levels, while the control group had a *decrease*. Helping people and showing kindness turns out to be good for *you* too.

So is gratitude. In a series of studies, psychologists found that those people who did things to cultivate feelings of gratitude, such as writing weekly journals, consistently felt happier and more optimistic.[28] Write down all the things you are grateful for in a gratitude journal at least once a week. You may be surprised with the length of the list. One experiment even showed that conveying gratitude can help us feel more relaxed. A group of volunteers was divided into three groups after being exposed to a standard stressor. The first group wrote an affectionate letter to a loved one, the second group simply thought about people they loved and why they loved them, and the others just sat quietly.[29] The results showed that stress levels among the letter-writing group *decreased* significantly while the thinking group had *increased* stress levels. In other words, it's not just thinking about a loved one that produces a positive response, but actually *conveying* that feeling. At the beginning of the study, the participants were asked to rate themselves on a scale that determined baseline affection. This baseline did not appear to make a difference in stress response, proving that even people who would not normally be affectionate can still experience the rewards of affection and gratitude.

Be grateful for your parents. Try not to get angry when they seem overbearing, because nobody else in the world is going to care for you as much. Since I first left home for university I have always called my parents every day to talk with them, even just for a couple of minutes. I have repeatedly encountered people who are shocked when I tell them this. "You really call your parents *every* day?" "How do you have the *time* for that?" My shock is that people don't! Your parents are the ones who brought you into the world, fed you when you were a helpless and dependent baby, and would stand by you through thick and thin. How can you not even give them a few minutes in your busy day? It's the least anyone can do.

While well-being goes hand in hand with happiness, the same does not necessarily apply to health. This may sound strange, because when we see all the illness and suffering around us, it should instantly give us some sense of perspective and gratitude. I remember once standing in a train station and seeing a young blind man walk through the foyer using his cane. A middle-aged lady stood beside me and said, "You know, that really helps put our own problems into perspective." How true. We often take our own health for granted and are none the happier for it. Unfortunately, physical health only appears to have an impact on our happiness levels when we are very ill.

Need something else to feel grateful for apart from food, warmth, health and family? You live in America and already have more than 95 percent of the world just by being here. It's likely that billions of people would trade positions with you in a heartbeat. You are also living at a great time. It's the 21st century and you have access to great technologies, medicines and life comforts that were not available to any other generation throughout history.

One of the most negative and self-defeating emotions you can harbor is jealousy or envy. It's depressing and a waste of time. The ironic thing about this emotion is that it actually sometimes arises for a good reason. We see something that we know we could have as well. Maybe we are underachieving or not working hard enough ourselves? Perhaps we know this deep inside and are just frustrated. It's natural, but don't get stuck on it or blame the other person. Make it about *yourself* instead. I recall reading a great article a few years ago about the uselessness of feeling envious of people who have more than you, especially with money. If there's something you want, then get to work on it, but green-eyed immobility is not a way forward. It won't make you richer, or the rich any poorer, but it will definitely make you sad and depressed! It should only be about what *you* can do to improve your own circumstances through self-reliance and hard work. Along the same lines, competition isn't necessarily a bad thing as long as it doesn't go over the top and become mean-spirited. We are built to be competitive, and it can be a potent driving force. This works on any level. Consider the space race between the United States and the former Soviet Union . Look how much was achieved in such a short time, sending people into space and then to the moon. How much have we really achieved since? Suppose for a minute that the race was still on. It's highly likely that we would have sent people to Mars and beyond by now! The positive benefits that can arise from competition shouldn't be underestimated.

Dreams are there to be had, but at the same time as you are pursuing them, you should never allow yourself to forget the pleasure of the moment. Rudyard Kipling said that you should be able to *dream, and not make dreams your master*. Goals and aspirations may be part of our well-being, but we shouldn't become so consumed by them that we forget the everyday simple pleasures. Whether we are talking about a first-year college student or a company president, there's unlikely to ever be a time when anyone can sit back and think, *That's it, I'm done*. The drive forward is continuous. And don't worry if you feel like you don't know exactly what you want. Few people do. It's the journey that counts.

Finally, when all is said and done, happiness will always remain a very subjective experience. Aristotle said that *happiness belongs more to those who have cultivated their character and mind to the uttermost.* Having just discussed the evidence regarding motivation, optimism and money, we can see how true this is. So can we summarize the enduring traits that happy people regularly exhibit? Absolutely. For a start, happy people pursue personal growth, always look on the bright side of life, and are the least materialistic. They don't dwell on unpleasant things and are able to move on quickly. They are grateful and aren't envious. They surround themselves with family and friends at every opportunity. We talked about getting *in the zone* a few chapters ago. Being able to absorb yourself in an activity that you enjoy and feel challenged by is one of the most rewarding experiences. Whether it is what you do at work, teaching, gardening or playing music—a life *in the zone* is likely to be a life of great satisfaction.

The best things in our lives that produce happiness are simultaneously free and priceless. They are also accessible at any moment, from spending time with family, seeing a loved one smile, watching the sunset or enjoying a simple stroll experiencing the awesome beauty of nature. There is, after all, so much happiness and well-being to be gained this very second.

HIGH PERCENTAGE LIFE STEPS

- Have the right motivation

    Focus on more intrinsic and less extrinsic reasons for your goals

- Avoid procrastination

    Make solid plans and tell those close to you

- Create a healthy relationship with money

    More money doesn't necessarily bring satisfaction and spending on experiences is better than spending on possessions

- Optimism and positivity affect your sense of well-being

    View your glass as half-full and not half-empty

- Expect obstacles

    Don't be put off by that first hurdle; some good can come out of setbacks

- Cultivate your mind for happiness

    Take on board those happiness traits

AFTERWORD

This book is quite personal to me. After graduating from medical school, like a lot of busy physicians, I went through a time when I slipped up and stopped caring for a while about my own health and wellness. With my hectic schedule, I wasn't taking proper care of what I was eating, didn't exercise regularly, started putting on weight and didn't participate in many hobbies outside of work. I also didn't have a set career path mapped out in my mind, and was uncertain for a time as to whether I was even in the right job! I found myself feeling more sluggish and tired, and started to dislike my occupation. Here I was fresh out of medical school in an extremely rewarding career that involved caring for other people, but not taking the right care of *myself*. I slowly began to realize that my lifestyle was contributing to my not feeling a true sense of well-being, and decided to take more charge of the situation. I made some much needed changes to my eating habits, activity levels, recreational pursuits and attitude. I began to think more about my own individual goals and increasingly absorbed myself in the parts of my work that I really enjoyed, while also trying to maintain a healthy work-life balance. Very soon, I started to feel much better and found that I was generally experiencing more life satisfaction. Many of the principles outlined in this book helped get me there!

We have gone through seven of the key pillars of wellness, and you've read about some natural, evidence-based steps that you can incorporate into your daily life. There's never going to be a magic formula that works for everyone, but taken together, the lifestyle changes we've gone over can help bring about dramatic improvements to your everyday well-being. To emphasize the point again, it's worth stating once more that many of the scientific studies included in this book have *higher* percentage changes beyond those at which new drugs are aggressively marketed. And that is the basic premise of this book…..that by adopting some simple easy habits, there can be a profound and long-lasting effect on your health. If eating more fruits, switching to whole grains, munching on a few walnuts, getting outdoors, spending time with friends, smiling and staying positive have been shown to do you so much good, imagine then what would happen if you did nine or ten good things. There will be a *cumulative* effect. The more of these healthy practices you adopt, the better it will be for you.

You must have noticed how a lot of the different concepts are interrelated and keep coming up again and again. Take exercise, for instance. It has benefits for weight loss, your mood and your energy levels. Drinking tea has anti-oxidant and stress-reducing properties. Eating low-glycemic foods can give you cardiovascular benefits as well as helping with your energy levels. Getting outdoors will give you exercise, invigorate you and also help you de-stress. Being optimistic brings more success, better health, and also helps with stress levels. The examples go on and on, with so many of these healthy habits intertwined.

We can view some of these wellness steps as a type of medicine too. Scientifically speaking, medicines are based on chemical molecules anyway. Instead of getting them in a pill, you are getting the great substances through an apple, blueberry or another fruit or vegetable instead. It's just getting into you more naturally. Other techniques like exercising, being with friends, or reading to improve mood and stress can also be thought of in this way too. Rather than taking a mood-boosting or relaxing medication, you are achieving the same brain effect via a more healthy method.

As I said in the introduction, modern medical advancements have been amazing and promoting well-being is not in any way a means of undermining all the great scientific advancements that are going on all around us. We can now cure previously incurable diseases through incredible new treatments and procedures. What you have read is simply about *lowering* your chances of illness arising in the first place. In other words, *prevention*. And even if you do have a medical condition, our bodies have an amazing propensity to replenish and reverse much of the damage if we adapt our lifestyles accordingly. It's never too late. If sickness strikes out of the blue, the chances of recovery are much better if your baseline health was built on solid foundations. This applies equally to minor ailments like the common cold or a sore throat, and to more serious conditions that require hospitalization.

Learning about all these wellness steps is one thing, and it's a good start to have the knowledge to go forward. But that's only the first part. The greater challenge is actually making sure you implement them. Remember, there's a difference between knowing the path and walking it. We can be told things many times, and even if we know inside it's true, actually doing it is a whole different ballgame. But the difference with health and well-being is this: When you give these lifestyle changes a chance, you are likely to quickly start *feeling* better. Your body will tell you that it likes healthy living, and this will be reflected in having a better body shape, improved mood, clearer mind and increased energy levels. You will feel so much better that you won't want to return to your old habits!

Your ultimate wealth is your health. So make a resolution to start right away. Begin with small steps. Make a conscious effort to eat more fruits and vegetables and consume only nonrefined carbohydrates. Leave an apple on your desk. Go low-glycemic. Take a brisk walk and use the stairs. Keep track of your weight. Get outdoors. Practice mental timeouts when you feel overwhelmed. Smile more. Stay optimistic. It is my hope that the wellness steps in this book can help you achieve more health and well-being in your life. I wish you the very best of luck.

ABOUT THE AUTHOR

Dr. Suneel Dhand, M.D. is board certified in Internal Medicine. He was born in London and grew up in Windsor, England. He went to medical school at Cardiff University, after which he moved across the pond to pursue further training, completing his internal medicine residency in Maryland. Seeing the tremendous opportunities for improvement, Suneel developed an interest in preventive medicine and wellness, which inspired him to write about the topic. *High Percentage Wellness Steps* is his first book.

REFERENCES

CHAPTER ONE

1. United States Department of Agriculture. *Agriculture Fact Book*, 2001-2002.

2. Weindruch R, Walford RL, Fligiel S, Guthrie D. The retardation of aging in mice by dietary restriction: longevity, cancer, immunity and lifetime energy intake. *Journal of Nutrition* 1986;116(4):641-54.

3. Liu S, Willett WC, Stampfer MJ, Hu FB, Franz M, Sampson L, Hennekens CH, Manson JE. A prospective study of dietary glycemic load, carbohydrate intake, and risk of coronary heart disease in US women. *American Journal of Clinical Nutrition* 2000;71(6):1455-61.

4. Hodge AM, English DR, O'Dea K, Giles GG. Glycemic index and dietary fiber and the risk of type 2 diabetes. *Diabetes Care* 2004;27(11):2701-6.

5. Tighe P, Duthie G, Vaughan N, Brittenden J, Simpson WG, Duthie S, Mutch W, Wahle K, Horgan G, Thies F. Effect of increased consumption of whole-grain foods on blood pressure and other cardiovascular risk markers in healthy middle-aged persons: a randomized controlled trial. *American Journal of Clinical Nutrition* 2010;92(4):733-40.

6. Sun Q, Spiegelman D, van Dam RM, Holmes MD, Malik VS, Willett WC, Hu FB. White rice, brown rice, and risk of type 2 diabetes in US men and women. *Archives of Internal Medicine* 2010;170(11):961-9.

7. Pereira MA, Jacobs DR Jr, Pins JJ, Raatz SK, Gross MD, Slavin JL, Seaquist ER. Effect of whole grains on insulin sensitivity in overweight hyperinsulinemic adults. *American Journal of Clinical Nutrition* 2002;75(5):848-55.

8. Peters U, Sinha R, Chatterjee N, Subar AF, Ziegler RG, Kulldorff M, Bresalier R, Weissfeld JL, Flood A, Schatzkin A, Hayes RB. Dietary fibre and colorectal adenoma in a colorectal cancer early detection programme. *Lancet* 2003;361(9368):1491-5.

9. Nomura AM, Hankin JH, Henderson BE, Wilkens LR, Murphy SP, Pike MC, Le Marchand L, Stram DO, Monroe KR, Kolonel LN. Dietary fiber and colorectal cancer risk: the multiethnic cohort study. *Cancer Causes and Control* 2007;18(7):753-64.

10. Park Y, Brinton LA, Subar AF, Hollenbeck A, Schatzkin A. Dietary fiber intake and risk of breast cancer in postmenopausal women: the National Institutes of Health-AARP Diet and Health Study. *American Journal of Clinical Nutrition* 2009;90(3):664-71.

11. Pelucchi C, Talamini R, Galeone C, Negri E, Franceschi S, Dal Maso L, Montella M, Conti E, La Vecchia C. Fibre intake and prostate cancer risk. *International Journal of Cancer* 2004;109(2):278-80.

12. *National Institutes of Health*, Bethesda, MD. 2011.

13. Sinha R, Cross AJ, Graubard BI, Leitzmann MF, Schatzkin A. Meat intake and mortality: a prospective study of over half a million people. *Archives of Internal Medicine* 2009;169(6):562-71.

14. Chao A, Thun MJ, Connell CJ, McCullough ML, Jacobs EJ, Flanders WD, Rodriguez C, Sinha R, Calle E. Meat consumption and risk of colorectal cancer. *Journal of the American Medical Association* 2005;293(2):172-82.

15. Norat T, Bingham S, Ferrari P et al. Meat, fish, and colorectal cancer risk: the European Prospective Investigation into cancer and nutrition. *Journal of the National Cancer Institute* 2005;97(12):906-16.

16. Ferrucci LM, Cross AJ, Graubard BI, Brinton LA, McCarty CA, Ziegler RG, Ma X, Mayne ST, Sinha R. Intake of meat, meat mutagens, and iron and the risk of breast cancer in the Prostate, Lung, Colorectal, and Ovarian Cancer Screening Trial. *British Journal of Cancer* 2009;101(1):178-84.

17. Chong EW, Simpson JA, Robman LD, Hodge AM, Aung KZ, English DR, Giles GG, Guymer RH. Red meat and chicken consumption and its association with age-related macular degeneration. *American Journal of Epidemiology* 2009;169(7):867-76.

18. Anderson JW, Johnstone BM, Cook-Newell ME. Meta-analysis of the effects of soy protein intake on serum lipids. *New England Journal of Medicine* 1995;333(5):276-82.

19. Mozaffarian D, Micha R, Wallace S. Effects on coronary heart disease of increasing polyunsaturated fat in place of saturated fat: a systematic review and meta-analysis of randomized controlled trials. *Public Library of Science Medicine* 2010; 23;7(3):e1000252.

20. Morris MC, Evans DA, Bienias JL, Tangney CC, Bennett DA, Aggarwal N, Schneider J, Wilson RS. Dietary fats and the risk of incident Alzheimer disease. *Archives of Neurology* 2003;60(2):194-200.

21. Mensink RP, Katan MB. Effect of dietary trans fatty acids on high-density and low-density lipoprotein cholesterol levels in healthy subjects. *New England Journal of Medicine* 1990;323(7):439-45.

22. *National Heart Foundation of Australia*, 2010.

23. Harnack L, Oakes M, French S, Cordy D, Montgomery M, Pettit J, King D. Trends in the fatty acid composition of frying oils used at leading fast food restaurants over the past 12 years based on french fries as a proxy indicator. *National Nutrient Database Conference* 2010; Grand Forks, ND.

24. Centers for Disease Control and Prevention. State-Specific Trends in Fruit and Vegetable Consumption Among Adults. *Behavioral Risk Factor Surveillance System*, 2000-2009.

25. Law MR, Morris JK. By how much does fruit and vegetable consumption reduce the risk of ischaemic heart disease? *European Journal of Clinical Nutrition* 1998;52(8):549-56.

26. Joshipura KJ, Hu FB, Manson JE, Stampfer MJ, Rimm EB, Speizer FE, Colditz G, Ascherio A, Rosner B, Spiegelman D, Willett WC. The effect of fruit and vegetable intake on risk for coronary heart disease. *Annals of Internal Medicine* 2001;134(12):1106-14.

27. Gillman MW, Cupples LA, Gagnon D, Posner BM, Ellison RC, Castelli WP, Wolf PA. Protective effect of fruits and vegetables on development of stroke in men. *Journal of the American Medical Association* 1995;273(14):1113-7.

28. Ford ES, Mokdad AH. Fruit and vegetable consumption and diabetes mellitus incidence among U.S. adults. *American Journal of Preventive Medicine* 2001;32(1):33-9.

29. Hung HC, Joshipura KJ, Jiang R, Hu FB, Hunter D, Smith-Warner SA, Colditz GA, Rosner B, Spiegelman D, Willett WC. Fruit and vegetable intake and risk of major chronic disease. *Journal of the National Cancer Institute* 2004;96(21):1577-84.

30. Hung HC, Willett W, Ascherio A, Rosner BA, Rimm E, Joshipura KJ. Tooth loss and dietary intake. *Journal of the American Dental Association* 2003;134(9):1185-92.

31. Gallus S, Talamini R, Giacosa A, Montella M, Ramazzotti V, Franceschi S, Negri E, La Vecchia C. Does an apple a day keep the oncologist away? *Annals of Oncology* 2005;16(11):1841-4.

32. Liu RH, Liu J, Chen B. Apples prevent mammary tumors in rats. *Journal of Agriculture and Food Chemistry* 2005;53(6):2341-3.

33. Eberhardt MV, Lee CY, Liu RH. Antioxidant activity of fresh apples. *Nature* 2000;405(6789):903-4.

34. Pearson DA, Tan CH, German JB, Davis PA, Gershwin ME. Apple juice inhibits human low density lipoprotein oxidation. *Life Sciences* 1999;64(21):1913-20.

35. Shaheen SO, Sterne JA, Thompson RL, Songhurst CE, Margetts BM, Burney PG. Dietary antioxidants and asthma in adults: population-based case-control study. *American Journal of Respiratory Critical Care Medicine* 2001;164(10):1823-8.

36. Butland BK, Fehily AM, Elwood PC. Diet, lung function, and lung function decline in a cohort of 2512 middle aged men. *Thorax* 2000;55(2):102-8.

37. Willers SM, Devereux G, Craig LC, McNeill G, Wijga AH, Abou El-Magd W, Turner SW, Helms PJ, Seaton A. Maternal food consumption during pregnancy and asthma, respiratory and atopic symptoms in 5-year-old children. *Thorax* 2007;62(9):773-9.

38. Papandreou MA, Dimakopoulou A, Linardaki ZI, Cordopatis P, Klimis-Zacas D, Margarity M, Lamari FN. Effect of a polyphenol-rich wild blueberry extract on cognitive performance of mice, brain antioxidant markers and acetylcholinesterase activity. *Behavioural Brain Research* 2009;198(2):352-8.

39. Poulose SM, Bielinski DF, Shukitt-Hale B, Fisher DR, Joseph JA. Berry extracts and brain aging: Clearance of toxic protein accumulation in brain via induction of autophagy. *American Chemical Society National Meeting* 2010; Boston, MA.

40. Basu A, Du M, Leyva MJ, Sanchez K, Betts NM, Wu M, Aston CE, Lyons TJ. Blueberries decrease cardiovascular risk factors in obese men and women with metabolic syndrome. *Journal of Nutrition* 2010;140(9):1582-7.

41. Stull AJ, Cash KC, Johnson WD, Champagne CM, Cefalu WT. Bioactives in blueberries improve insulin sensitivity in obese, insulin-resistant men and women. *Journal of Nutrition* 2010;140(10):1764-8.

42. Sabaté J, Oda K, Ros E. Nut consumption and blood lipid levels: a pooled analysis of 25 intervention trials. *Archives of Internal Medicine* 2010;170(9):821-7.

43. Banel DK, Hu FB. Effects of walnut consumption on blood lipids and other cardiovascular risk factors: a meta-analysis and systematic review. *American Journal of Clinical Nutrition* 2009;90(1):56-63.

44. Jenkins DJ, Kendall CW, Marchie A, Parker TL, Connelly PW, Qian W, Haight JS, Faulkner D, Vidgen E, Lapsley KG, Spiller GA. Dose response of almonds on coronary heart disease risk factors: blood lipids, oxidized low-density lipoproteins, lipoprotein(a), homocysteine, and pulmonary nitric oxide: a randomized, controlled, crossover trial. *Circulation* 2002;106(11):1327-32.

45. Bibbins-Domingo K, Chertow GM, Coxson PG, Moran A, Lightwood JM, Pletcher MJ, Goldman L. Projected effect of dietary salt reductions on future cardiovascular disease. *New England Journal of Medicine* 2010;362(7):590-9.

46. Jenkins DJ, Kendall CW, Marchie A, Jenkins AL, Augustin LS, Ludwig DS, Barnard ND, Anderson JW. Type 2 diabetes and the vegetarian diet. *American Journal of Clinical Nutrition* 2003;78(3):610S-616S.

47. Key TJ, Appleby PN, Travis RC, Allen NE, Thorogood M, Mann JI. Cancer incidence in British vegetarians. *British Journal of Cancer* 2009;101:192–197.

48. Sabaté J, Wien M. Vegetarian diets and childhood obesity prevention. *American Journal of Clinical Nutrition* 2010;91(5):1525S-1529S.

49. Gale CR, Deary IJ, Schoon I, Batty GD. IQ in childhood and vegetarianism in adulthood: 1970 British cohort study. *British Medical Journal* 2007;334(7587):245.

50. Fung TT, van Dam RM, Hankinson SE, Stampfer M, Willett WC, Hu FB. Low-carbohydrate diets and all-cause and cause-specific mortality: two cohort studies. *Annals of Internal Medicine* 2010;153(5):289-98.

51. Janszky I, Mukamal KJ, Ljung R, Ahnve S, Ahlbom A, Hallqvist J. Chocolate consumption and mortality following a first acute myocardial infarction: the Stockholm Heart Epidemiology Program. *Journal of Internal Medicine* 2009;266(3):248-57.

52. Lewis JR, Prince RL, Zhu K, Devine A, Thompson PL, Hodgson JM. Habitual chocolate intake and vascular disease: a prospective study of clinical outcomes in older women. *Archives of Internal Medicine* 2010;170(20):1857-8.

53. Sofi F, Cesari F, Abbate R, Gensini GF, Casini A. Adherence to Mediterranean diet and health status: meta-analysis. *British Medical Journal* 2008;337:a1344.

54. The Importance of Family Dinners VI. *National Center on Addiction and Substance Abuse at Columbia University,* 2010.

CHAPTER TWO

1. Ruiz JR, Sui X, Lobelo F, Morrow JR Jr, Jackson AW, Sjöström M, Blair SN. Association between muscular strength and mortality in men: prospective cohort study. *British Medical Journal* 2008;337(7661):92–95.

2. Tanasescu M, Leitzmann MF, Rimm EB, Willett WC, Stampfer MJ, Hu FB. Exercise type and intensity in relation to coronary heart disease in men. *Journal of the American Medical Association* 2002;288(16):1994-2000.

3. Sandvik L, Erikssen J, Thaulow E, Erikssen G, Mundal R, Rodahl K. Physical fitness as a predictor of mortality among healthy, middle-aged Norwegian men. *New England Journal of Medicine* 1993;328(8):533-7.

4. Manson JE, Hu FB, Rich-Edwards JW, Colditz GA, Stampfer MJ, Willett WC, Speizer FE, Hennekens CH. A prospective study of walking as compared with vigorous exercise in the prevention of coronary heart disease in women. *New England Journal of Medicine* 1999;341(9):650-8.

5. Lee IM, Rexrode KM, Cook NR, Manson JE, Buring JE. Physical activity and coronary heart disease in women: is "no pain, no gain" passé? *Journal of the American Medical Association* 2001;285(11):1447-54.

6. Paffenbarger RS Jr, Hyde RT, Wing AL, Lee IM, Jung DL, Kampert JB. The association of changes in physical-activity level and other lifestyle characteristics with mortality among men. *New England Journal of Medicine* 1993;328(8):538-45.

7. Steffen-Batey L, Nichaman MZ, Goff DC Jr, Frankowski RF, Hanis CL, Ramsey DJ, Labarthe DR. Change in level of physical activity and risk of all-cause mortality or reinfarction: The Corpus Christi Heart Project. *Circulation* 2000;102(18):2204-9.

8. Wannamethee SG, Shaper AG, Walker M. Physical activity and mortality in older men with diagnosed coronary heart disease. *Circulation* 2000;102(12):1358-63.

9. Palatini P, Visentin P, Dorigatti F, Guarnieri C, Santonastaso M, Cozzio S, Pegoraro F, Bortolazzi A, Vriz O, Mos L. Regular physical activity prevents development of left ventricular hypertrophy in hypertension. *European Heart Journal* 2009;30(2):225-32.

10. Hakim AA, Curb JD, Petrovitch H, Rodriguez BL, Yano K, Ross GW, White LR, Abbott RD. Effects of walking on coronary heart disease in elderly men: the Honolulu Heart Program. *Circulation* 1999;100(1):9-13.

11. Hakim AA, Petrovitch H, Burchfiel CM, Ross GW, Rodriguez BL, White LR, Yano K, Curb JD, Abbott RD. Effects of walking on mortality among nonsmoking retired men. *New England Journal of Medicine* 1998;338(2):94-9.

12. Zullig KJ, White RJ. Physical Activity, Life Satisfaction, and Self-Rated Health of Middle School Students. *Applied Research in Quality of Life* 2010;DOI:10.1007/s11482-010-9129-z.

13. Hu FB, Sigal RJ, Rich-Edwards JW, Colditz GA, Solomon CG, Willett WC, Speizer FE, Manson JE. Walking compared with vigorous physical activity and risk of type 2 diabetes in women: a prospective study. *Journal of the American Medical Association* 1999;282(15):1433-9.

14. Kampert JB, Blair SN, Barlow CE, Kohl HW 3rd. Physical activity, physical fitness, and all-cause and cancer mortality: a prospective study of men and women. *Annals of Epidemiology* 1996;6(5):452-7.

15. Eliassen AH, Hankinson SE, Rosner B, Holmes MD, Willett WC. Physical activity and risk of breast cancer among postmenopausal women. *Archives of Internal Medicine* 2010;170(19):1758-64.

16. Peel JB, Sui X, Adams SA, Hébert JR, Hardin JW, Blair SN. A prospective study of cardiorespiratory fitness and breast cancer mortality. *Medicine & Science in Sports & Exercise* 2009;41(4):742-8.

17. Korpelainen R, Keinänen-Kiukaanniemi S, Nieminen P, Heikkinen J, Väänänen K, Korpelainen J. Long-term outcomes of exercise: follow-up of a randomized trial in older women with osteopenia. *Archives of Internal Medicine* 2010;170(17):1548-56.

18. Hu G, Eriksson J, Barengo NC, Lakka TA, Valle TT, Nissinen A, Jousilahti P, Tuomilehto J. Occupational, commuting, and leisure-time physical activity in relation to total and cardiovascular mortality among Finnish subjects with type 2 diabetes. *Circulation* 2004;110(6):666-73.

19. Blumenthal JA, Babyak MA, Moore KA, Craighead WE, Herman S, Khatri P, Waugh R, Napolitano MA, Forman LM, Appelbaum M, Doraiswamy PM, Krishnan KR. Effects of exercise training on older patients with major depression. *Archives of Internal Medicine* 1999;159(19):2349-56.

20. Babyak M, Blumenthal JA, Herman S, Khatri P, Doraiswamy M, Moore K, Craighead WE, Baldewicz TT, Krishnan KR. Exercise treatment for major depression: maintenance of therapeutic benefit at 10 months. *Psychosomatic Medicine* 2000;62(5):633-8.

21. Blumenthal JA, Babyak MA, Doraiswamy PM, Watkins L, Hoffman BM, Barbour KA, Herman S, Craighead WE, Brosse AL, Waugh R, Hinderliter A, Sherwood A. Exercise and pharmacotherapy in the treatment of major depressive disorder. *Psychosomatic Medicine* 2007;69(7):587-96.

22. Steinberg H, Sykes EA, Moss T, Lowery S, LeBoutillier N, Dewey A. Exercise enhances creativity independently of mood. *British Journal of Sports Medicine* 1997;31(3):240-5.

23. Lane AM, Lovejoy DJ. The effects of exercise on mood changes: the moderating effect of depressed mood. *Journal of Sports Medicine and Physical Fitness* 2001;41(4):539-45.

24. Flynn J, Ode J. Hit the treadmill – not just the books – to boost grades. *American College of Sports Medicine Annual Meeting* 2010; Baltimore, MD.

25. Aberg MA, Pedersen NL, Torén K, Svartengren M, Bäckstrand B, Johnsson T, Cooper-Kuhn CM, Aberg ND, Nilsson M, Kuhn HG. Cardiovascular fitness is associated with cognition in young adulthood. *Proceedings of the National Academy of Sciences of the United States of America* 2009;106(49):20906-11.

26. Erickson KI, Raji CA, Lopez OL, Becker JT, Rosano C, Newman AB, Gach HM, Thompson PM, Ho AJ, Kuller LH. Physical activity predicts gray matter volume in late adulthood: the Cardiovascular Health Study. *Neurology* 2010;75(16):1415-22.

27. Erickson KI, Voss MW, Prakash RS et al. Exercise training increases size of hippocampus and improves memory. *Proceedings of the National Academy of Sciences of the United States of America* 2011;108(7):3017-22.

28. Hagberg LA, Lindahl B, Nyberg L, Hellénius ML. Importance of enjoyment when promoting physical exercise. *Scandinavian Journal of Medicine & Science in Sports* 2009;19(5):740-7.

CHAPTER THREE

1. Finucane MM, Stevens GA, Cowan MJ et al. National, regional, and global trends in body-mass index since 1980: systematic analysis of health examination surveys and epidemiological studies with 960 country-years and 9·1 million participants. *Lancet* 2011;377(9765):557-67.

2. Ogden CL, Carroll MD. Prevalence of Obesity Among Children and Adolescents: United States, Trends 1963–1965 Through 2007–2008. *Centers for Disease Control and Prevention*, 2010.

3. Wang Y, Beydoun MA, Liang L, Caballero B, Kumanyika SK. Will all Americans become overweight or obese? Estimating the progression and cost of the US obesity epidemic. *Obesity* 2008;16(10):2323-30.

4. Behan, DF, Cox SH, Lin Y, Pai J, Pedersen HW and Yi M Obesity and its Relation to Mortality and Morbidity Costs. *Society of Actuaries*, 2010.

5. Bish CL, Blanck HM, Serdula MK, Marcus M, Kohl HW 3rd, Khan LK. Diet and physical activity behaviors among Americans trying to lose weight: 2000 Behavioral Risk Factor Surveillance System. *Obesity Research* 2005;13(3):596-607.

6. Wannamethee SG, Shaper AG, Walker M. Overweight and obesity and weight change in middle aged men: impact on cardiovascular disease and diabetes. *Journal of Epidemiology & Community Health* 2005;59(2):134-9.

7. Harris Poll. *Harris Interactive*, 2011.

8. Abid A, Galuska D, Khan LK, Gillespie C, Ford ES, Serdula MK. Are healthcare professionals advising obese patients to lose weight? A trend analysis. *Medscape General Medicine* 2005;7(4):10.

9. Ajani UA, Lotufo PA, Gaziano JM, Lee IM, Spelsberg A, Buring JE, Willett WC, Manson JE. Body mass index and mortality among US male physicians. *Annals of Epidemiology* 2004;14(10):731-9.

10. Dobbelsteyn CJ, Joffres MR, MacLean DR, Flowerdew G. A comparative evaluation of waist circumference, waist-to-hip ratio and body mass index as indicators of cardiovascular risk factors. The Canadian Heart Health Surveys. *International Journal of Obesity and Related Metabolic Disorders* 2001;25(5):652-61.

11. Wei M, Gaskill SP, Haffner SM, Stern MP. Waist circumference as the best predictor of noninsulin dependent diabetes mellitus (NIDDM) compared to body mass index, waist/hip ratio and other anthropometric measurements in Mexican Americans—a 7-year prospective study. *Obesity Research* 1997;5(1):16-23.

12. Rozmus-Wrzesinska M, Pawlowski B. Men's ratings of female attractiveness are influenced more by changes in female waist size compared with changes in hip size. *Biological Psychology* 2005;68(3):299-308.

13. Gardner CD, Kiazand A, Alhassan S, Kim S, Stafford RS, Balise RR, Kraemer HC, King AC. Comparison of the Atkins, Zone, Ornish, and LEARN diets for change in weight and related risk factors among overweight premenopausal women: the A TO Z Weight Loss Study: a randomized trial. *Journal of the American Medical Association* 2007;297(9):969-77.

14. Foster GD, Wyatt HR, Hill JO et al. Weight and metabolic outcomes after 2 years on a low-carbohydrate versus low-fat diet: a randomized trial. *Annals of Internal Medicine* 2010;153(3):147-57.

15. Sacks FM, Bray GA, Carey VJ et al. Comparison of weight-loss diets with different compositions of fat, protein, and carbohydrates. *New England Journal of Medicine* 2009;360(9):859-73.

16. Johnstone AM, Horgan GW, Murison SD, Bremner DM, Lobley GE. Effects of a high-protein ketogenic diet on hunger, appetite, and weight loss in obese men feeding ad libitum. *American Journal of Clinical Nutrition* 2008;87(1):44-55.

17. Dennis EA, Dengo AL, Comber DL, Flack KD, Savla J, Davy KP, Davy BM. Water consumption increases weight loss during a hypocaloric diet intervention in middle-aged and older adults. *Obesity* 2010;18(2):300-7.

18. Stookey JD, Constant F, Popkin BM, Gardner CD. Drinking water is associated with weight loss in overweight dieting women independent of diet and activity. *Obesity* 2008;16(11):2481-8.

19. Mandal B. Use of Food Labels as a Weight Loss Behavior. *Journal of Consumer Affairs* 2010;44(3):516–527.

20. Hollis JF, Gullion CM, Stevens VJ et al. Weight loss during the intensive intervention phase of the weight-loss maintenance trial. *American Journal of Preventive Medicine* 2008;35(2):118-26.

21. Sentyrz SM, Bushman BJ. Mirror, mirror on the wall, who's the thinnest one of all? Effects of self-awareness on consumption of full-fat, reduced-fat, and no-fat products. *Journal of Applied Psychology* 1998;83(6):944-9.

22. Morewedge CK, Huh YE, Vosgerau J. Thought for food: imagined consumption reduces actual consumption. *Science* 2010;330(6010):1530-3.

23. Kapinos KA, Yakusheva O. Environmental influences on young adult weight gain: evidence from a natural experiment. *Journal of Adolescent Health* 2011;48(1):52-8.

24. Racette SB, Weiss EP, Schechtman KB, Steger-May K, Villareal DT, Obert KA, Holloszy JO. Influence of weekend lifestyle patterns on body weight. *Obesity* 2008;16(8):1826-30.

25. Delmas C, Platat C, Schweitzer B, Wagner A, Oujaa M, Simon C. Association between television in bedroom and adiposity throughout adolescence. *Obesity* 2007;15(10):2495-503.

26. McGuire MT, Wing RR, Klem ML, Lang W, Hill JO. What predicts weight regain in a group of successful weight losers? *Journal of Consulting and Clinical Psychology* 1999;67(2):177-85.

27. Phelan S, Liu T, Gorin A, Lowe M, Hogan J, Fava J, Wing RR. What distinguishes weight-loss maintainers from the treatment-seeking obese? Analysis of environmental, behavioral, and psychosocial variables in diverse populations. *Annals of Behavioral Medicine* 2009;38(2):94-104.

28. Kruger J, Blanck HM, Gillespie C. Dietary and physical activity behaviors among adults successful at weight loss maintenance. *International Journal of Behavioural Nutrition and Physical Activity* 2006;3:17.

29. Webber KH, Tate DF, Ward DS, Bowling JM. Motivation and its relationship to adherence to self-monitoring and weight loss in a 16-week Internet behavioral weight loss intervention. *Journal of Nutrition Education and Behavior* 2010;42(3):161-7.

30. Linde JA, Erickson DJ, Jeffery RW, Pronk NP, Boyle RG. The relationship between prevalence and duration of weight loss strategies and weight loss among overweight managed care organization members enrolled in a weight loss trial. *International Journal of Behavioural Nutrition and Physical Activity* 2006;17;3:3.

31. Schlundt DG, Hill JO, Sbrocco T, Pope-Cordle J, Sharp T. The role of breakfast in the treatment of obesity: a randomized clinical trial. *American Journal of Clinical Nutrition* 1992;55(3):645-51.

CHAPTER FOUR

1. Cullen W, Kearney Y, Bury G. Prevalence of fatigue in general practice. *Irish Journal of Medical Sciences* 2002;171(1):10-2.

2. Mengel MB, Schwiebert LP, eds. *Family Medicine: Ambulatory Care & Prevention*, 4th edition. New York: McGraw-Hill, 2005.

3. Holt SH, Delargy HJ, Lawton CL, Blundell JE. The effects of high carbohydrate vs high-fat breakfasts on feelings of fullness and alertness, and subsequent food intake. *International Journal of Food Sciences & Nutrition* 1999;50(1):13-28.

4. Handley R, Dye L, King N. Effect of meals varying in macronutrient composition and Glycaemic Index on mental performance, mood and appetite. *Proceedings of the British Psychological Society* 2003;11(2):271-72.

5. Anderson C, Horne JA. A high sugar content, low caffeine drink does not alleviate sleepiness but may worsen it. *Human Psychopharmacology: Clinical & Experimental* 2006;21(5):299-303.

6. Ryan RM, Weinstein N, Bernstein J, Brown KW, Mistretta L, Gagne M. Vitalizing effects of being outdoors and in nature. *Journal of Environmental Psychology* 2010;30(2):159–168.

7. Keller, M. C., Fredrickson, B. L., Ybarra, O., Cote, S., Johnson, K., Mikels, J., Conway, A., & Wager, T. A warm heart and a clear head: The contingent effects of weather on human mood and cognition. *Psychological Science* 2005;16(9):724-731.

8. Etcoff, N. The home ecology of flowers. *Harvard University*, 2006.

9. Pronin E, Wegner DM. Manic thinking: independent effects of thought speed and thought content on mood. *Psychological Science* 2006;17(9):807-13.

10. Pronin E, Jacobs E, Wegner DM. Psychological effects of thought acceleration. *Emotion* 2008;8(5):597-612.

11. Balci R,Aghazadeh F. Effects of exercise breaks on performance, muscular load, and perceived discomfort in data entry and cognitive tasks. *Computers & Industrial Engineering* 2004;46(3):399-411.

12. Puetz TW, O'Connor PJ, Dishman RK. Effects of chronic exercise on feelings of energy and fatigue: a quantitative synthesis. *Psychological Bulletin* 2006;132(6):866-76.

13. Thayer, RE, Biakanja L, O'Hanian P, Sorrell KAT, Balasanian A, Clemens AS, Fasi JO. Amount of Daily Walking Predicts Energy, Mood, Personality, and Health. *American Psychological Association Annual Convention* 2005; Washington, DC.

14. Thayer RE. Energy, tiredness, and tension effects of a sugar snack versus moderate exercise. *Journal of Personality and Social Psychology* 1987;52(1):119-25.

15. Sleep in America Poll. *National Sleep Foundation*, 2010.

16. Cappuccio FP, Stranges S, Kandala NB, Miller MA, Taggart FM, Kumari M, Ferrie JE, Shipley MJ, Brunner EJ, Marmot MG. Gender-specific associations of short sleep duration with prevalent and incident hypertension: the Whitehall II Study. *Hypertension* 2007;50(4):693-700.

17. Gangwisch JE, Heymsfield SB, Boden-Albala B, Buijs RM, Kreier F, Pickering TG, Rundle AG, Zammit GK, Malaspina D. Short sleep duration as a risk factor for hypertension: analyses of the first National Health and Nutrition Examination Survey. *Hypertension* 2006;47(5):833-9.

18. Glozier N, Martiniuk A, Patton G, Ivers R, Li Q, Hickie I, Senserrick T, Woodward M, Norton R, Stevenson M. Short sleep duration in prevalent and persistent psychological distress in young adults: the DRIVE study. *Sleep* 2010;33(9):1139-45.

19. Chang PP, Ford DE, Mead LA, Cooper-Patrick L, Klag MJ. Insomnia in young men and subsequent depression. The Johns Hopkins Precursors Study. *American Journal of Epidemiology* 1997;146(2):105-14.

20. Szklo-Coxe M, Young T, Peppard PE, Finn LA, Benca RM. Prospective associations of insomnia markers and symptoms with depression. *American Journal of Epidemiology* 2010;171(6):709-20.

21. Cappuccio FP, D'Elia L, Strazzullo P, Miller MA. Sleep duration and all-cause mortality: a systematic review and meta-analysis of prospective studies. *Sleep* 2010;33(5):585-92.

22. Nedeltcheva AV, Kilkus JM, Imperial J, Schoeller DA, Penev PD. Insufficient sleep undermines dietary efforts to reduce adiposity. *Annals of Internal Medicine* 2010;153(7):435-41.

CHAPTER FIVE

1. Stress in America. *American Psychological Association*, 2010.

2. Stress in America. *American Psychological Association*, 2007.

3. *Integra Realty Resources, Inc. Survey*, 2000.

4. Pryor JH, Hurtado S, DeAngelo L, Palucki Blake L, Tran S. The American Freshman: National Norms for Fall 2010. *Higher Education Research Institute. University of California, Los Angeles*, 2011.

5. *The American Institute of Stress*, NY. 2004.

6. Vogelzangs N, Beekman AT, Milaneschi Y, Bandinelli S, Ferrucci L, Penninx BW. Urinary cortisol and six-year risk of all-cause and cardiovascular mortality. *Journal of Clinical Endocrinology & Metabolism* 2010;95(11):4959-64.

7. Chen Y, Rex CS, Rice CJ, Dubé CM, Gall CM, Lynch G, Baram TZ. Correlated memory defects and hippocampal dendritic spine loss after acute stress involve corticotropin-releasing hormone signaling. *Proceedings of the National Academy of Sciences of the United States of America* 2010;107(29):13123-8.

8. Tottenham N, Hare TA, Quinn BT et al. Prolonged institutional rearing is associated with atypically large amygdala volume and difficulties in emotion regulation. *Developmental Science* 2010;13(1):46-61.

9. Tang YY, Ma Y, Wang J, Fan Y, Feng S, Lu Q, Yu Q, Sui D, Rothbart MK, Fan M, Posner MI. Short-term meditation training improves attention and self-regulation. *Proceedings of the National Academy of Sciences of the United States of America* 2007;104(43):17152-6.

10. Kabat-Zinn J, Massion AO, Kristeller J, Peterson LG, Fletcher KE, Pbert L, Lenderking WR, Santorelli SF. Effectiveness of a meditation-based stress reduction program in the treatment of anxiety disorders. *American Journal of Psychiatry* 1992;149(7):936-43.

11. Kabat-Zinn, J., Lipworth, L., Burney, R. and Sellers, W. Four year follow-up of a meditation-based program for the self-regulation of chronic pain: Treatment outcomes and compliance. *Clinical Journal of Pain* 1986 2(3):159-174.

12. Grossman P, Kappos L, Gensicke H, D'Souza M, Mohr DC, Penner IK, Steiner C. MS quality of life, depression, and fatigue improve after mindfulness training: a randomized trial. *Neurology* 2010;75(13):1141-9.

13. Nawijn J, Marchand MA, Veenhoven R, Vingerhoets AJ. Vacationers Happier, but Most not Happier After a Holiday. *Applied Research in Quality of Life* 2010;5(1):35-47.

14. Westman M, Eden D. Effects of a respite from work on burnout: vacation relief and fade-out. *Journal of Applied Psychology* 1997;82(4):516-27.

15. Allen K, Shykoff BE, Izzo JL Jr. Pet ownership, but not ace inhibitor therapy, blunts home blood pressure responses to mental stress. *Hypertension* 2001;38(4):815-20.

16. Allen K, Blascovich J, Mendes WB. Cardiovascular reactivity and the presence of pets, friends, and spouses: the truth about cats and dogs. *Psychosomatic Medicine* 2002;64(5):727-39.

17. Friedmann E, Thomas SA. Pet ownership, social support, and one-year survival after acute myocardial infarction in the Cardiac Arrhythmia Suppression Trial (CAST). *American Journal of Cardiology* 1995;76(17):1213-7.

18. Siegel JM. Stressful life events and use of physician services among the elderly: the moderating role of pet ownership. *Journal of Personality and Social Psychology* 1990;58(6):1081-6.

19. Raina P, Waltner-Toews D, Bonnett B, Woodward C, Abernathy T. Influence of companion animals on the physical and psychological health of older people: an analysis of a one-year longitudinal study. *Journal of American Geriatrics Society* 1999;47(3):323-9.

20. Wells M, Perrine R. Critters in the cube farm: perceived psychological and organizational effects of pets in the workplace. *Journal of Occupational Health Psychology* 2001;6(1):81-7.

21. Pup-Peroni. New Wags, Not Words Survey. *Kelton Research*, 2000.

22. Steptoe A, Gibson EL, Vuononvirta R, Williams ED, Hamer M, Rycroft JA, Erusalimsky JD, Wardle J. The effects of tea on psychophysiological stress responsivity and post-stress recovery: a randomised double-blind trial. *Psychopharmacology* 2007;190(1):81-9.

23. Melnick M. Study: A Handful of Walnuts a Day May Help Keep Stress Away. Study by West SG, Pennsylvania State University. *Time* October 2010.

24. *Mindlab International Ltd. University of Sussex*, 2009.

25. Lambiase MJ, Barry HM, Roemmich JN. Effect of a simulated active commute to school on cardiovascular stress reactivity. *Medicine & Science in Sports & Exercise* 2010;42(8):1609-16.

CHAPTER SIX

1. Willis J, Todorov A. First impressions: making up your mind after a 100-ms exposure to a face. *Psychological Science* 2006;17(7):592-8.

2. Ballew CC 2nd, Todorov A. Predicting political elections from rapid and unreflective face judgments. *Proceedings of the National Academy of Sciences of the United States of America* 2007;104(46):17948-53.

3. Stewart GL, Dustin SL, Barrick MR, Darnold TC. Exploring the handshake in employment interviews. *Journal of Applied Psychology* 2008;93(5):1139-46.

4. Farroni T, Csibra G, Simion F, Johnson MH. Eye contact detection in humans from birth. *Proceedings of the National Academy of Sciences of the United States of America* 2002;99(14):9602-5.

5. Wang Y, Newport R, Hamilton AF. Eye contact enhances mimicry of intransitive hand movements. *Biology Letters* 2011;7(1):7-10.

6. Farroni T, Menon E, Rigato S, Johnson MH. The perception of facial expressions in newborns. *European Journal of Developmental Psychology* 2007;4(1):2-13.

7. Haidt J, Keltner D. Culture and Facial Expression: Open-ended Methods Find More Expressions and a Gradient of Recognition. *Cognition & Emotion* 1999;13(3):225-266.

8. Soussignan R. Duchenne smile, emotional experience, and autonomic reactivity: a test of the facial feedback hypothesis. *Emotion* 2002;2(1):52-74.

9. Schnall S, Laird JD. Keep smiling: Enduring effects of facial expressions and postures on emotional experience and memory. *Cognition and Emotion* 2003;17(5):787-797.

10. Scharlemann, J.P.W., Eckel, C.C., Kacelnik, A. & Wilson, R.K. The value of a smile: game theory with a human face. *Journal of Economic Psychology* 2001;22(5): 617-640.

11. Surakka V, Hietanen JK. Facial and emotional reactions to Duchenne and non-Duchenne smiles. *International Journal of Psychophysiology* 1998;29(1):23-33.

12. Scott BA, Barnes CM. A Multilevel Field Investigation of Emotional Labor, Affect, Work Withdrawal, and Gender. *Academy of Management Journal* 2011;54 (1):116-136.

13. Hertenstein M, Hansel C, Butts A, & Hile S. Smile intensity in photographs predicts divorce later in life. *Motivation and Emotion* 2009;DOI 10.1007/s11031-009-9124-6.

14. Abel EL, Kruger ML. Smile intensity in photographs predicts longevity. *Psychological Science* 2010;21(4):542-4.

15. Seiter JS, Weger H Jr. The Effect of Generalized Compliments, Sex of Server, and Size of Dining Party on Tipping Behavior in Restaurants. *Journal of Applied Social Psychology* 2010;40:(1)1-12.

16. Seiter JS, Dutson E. The Effect of Compliments on Tipping Behavior in Hairstyling Salons. *Journal of Applied Social Psychology* 2007;37(9):1999–2007.

17. Bernstein E. I'm Very, Very, Very Sorry...Really? *Wall Street Journal* October 2010.

18. Schumann K, Ross M. Why women apologize more than men: gender differences in thresholds for perceiving offensive behavior. *Psychological Science* 2010;21(11):1649-55.

19. Carney DR, Cuddy AJ, Yap AJ. Power Posing: Brief Nonverbal Displays Affect Neuroendocrine Levels and Risk Tolerance *Psychological Science* 2010;21(10):1363-8.

20. Casciaro T, Lobo MS. Competent jerks, lovable fools, and the formation of social networks. *Harvard Business Review* 2005;83(6):92-9.

21. Seiter JS, Weger H Jr. Audience perceptions of candidates' appropriateness as a function of nonverbal behaviors displayed during televised political debates. *Journal of Social Psychology* 2005;145(2):225-35.

22. Yuill N, Ruffman T. The Relation Between Parenting, Children's Social Understanding and Language. *Economic and Social Research Council*, 2009.

23. Giles LC, Glonek GF, Luszcz MA, Andrews GR. Effect of social networks on 10 year survival in very old Australians: the Australian longitudinal study of aging. *Journal of Epidemiology & Community Health* 2005;59(7):574-9.

24. Holt-Lunstad J, Smith TB, Layton JB. Social relationships and mortality risk: a meta-analytic review. *Public Library of Science Medicine* 2010;7(7):e1000316.

25. *National Opinion Research Center. University of Chicago.*

26. Stack S, Eshleman JR. Marital Status and Happiness: A 17-Nation Study *Journal of Marriage and Family* 1998;60(2):527-536.

27. Headey B, Muffels R, Wagner GG. Long-running German panel survey shows that personal and economic choices, not just genes, matter for happiness. *Proceedings of the National Academy of Sciences of the United States of America* 2010;107(42):17922-6.

28. Wild B, Erb M, Bartels M. Are emotions contagious? Evoked emotions while viewing emotionally expressive faces: quality, quantity, time course and gender differences. *Psychiatry Research* 2001;102(2):109-24.

29. Hill AL, Rand DG, Nowak MA, Christakis NA. Emotions as infectious diseases in a large social network: the SISa model. *Proceedings of the Royal Society Biological Sciences* 2010;277(1701):3827-35.

30. Fowler JH, Christakis NA. Dynamic spread of happiness in a large social network: longitudinal analysis over 20 years in the Framingham Heart Study. *British Medical Journal* 2008;337:a2338.

31. Capitalizing on Effective Communication. How Courage, Innovation and Discipline Drive Business Results in Challenging Times. 2009/2010 Communication ROI Study Report. *Watson Wyatt Worldwide*, 2010.

32. The Return on Investment of US Business Travel. *Oxford Economics USA*. September 2009.

CHAPTER SEVEN

1. Lyubomirsky S, King L, Diener E. The benefits of frequent positive affect: does happiness lead to success? *Psychological Bulletin* 2005;131(6):803-55.

2. Amabile TM. Motivation and Creativity: Effects of Motivational Orientation on Creative Writers. *Journal of Personality and Social Psychology* 1985;48(2):393-399.

3. Lepper MR, Greene D, Nisbett RE. Undermining children's intrinsic interest with extrinsic reward: a test of the "overjustification" hypothesis *Journal of Personality and Social Psychology* 1973;28(1):129-137.

4. Niemiec CP, Ryan RM, Deci EL. The Path Taken: Consequences of Attaining Intrinsic and Extrinsic Aspirations in Post-College Life. *Journal of Research in Personality* 2009;73(3):291-306.

5. Steel P. The nature of procrastination: a meta-analytic and theoretical review of quintessential self-regulatory failure. *Psychological Bulletin* 2007;133(1):65-94.

6. Matthews G. Goals Research Study. *Dominican University of California*, 2007.

7. Kahneman D, Deaton A. High income improves evaluation of life but not emotional well-being. *Proceedings of the National Academy of Sciences of the United States of America* 2010;107(38):16489–16493.

8. Boyce CJ, Brown GD, Moore SC. Money and happiness: rank of income, not income, affects life satisfaction. *Psychological Science* 2010;21(4):471-5.

9. Zink CF, Pagnoni G, Martin-Skurski ME, Chappelow JC, Berns GS. Human striatal responses to monetary reward depend on saliency. *Neuron* 2004;42(3):509-17.

10. Howell RT, Hill G. The mediators of experiential purchases: Determining the impact of psychological needs satisfaction and social comparison. *Journal of Positive Psychology* 2009;4(6):511-522.

11. Harris Interactive Survey. *Northwestern Mutual Financial Network*, 2003.

12. Seligman MEP, Schulman P. Explanatory Style as a Predictor of Productivity and Quitting Among Life Insurance Sales Agents. *Journal of Personality and Social Psychology* 1986;50(4):832-838.

13. Williams G. Links Between Optimism-Building and Problem Solving Capacity. *International Congress on Mathematical Education* 2008; Monterrey, Mexico.

14. Williams G. How Group Composition Can Influence Opportunities for Spontaneous Learning. *Proceedings of the 31st Annual Conference of the Mathematics Education Research Group of Australasia* 2008:581-88.

15. Delbaere K, Close JC, Brodaty H, Sachdev P, Lord SR. Determinants of disparities between perceived and physiological risk of falling among elderly people: cohort study. *British Medical Journal* 2010;341:c4165.

16. Danner DD, Snowdon DA, Friesen WV. Positive emotions in early life and longevity: findings from the nun study. *Journal of Personality and Social Psychology.* 2001;80(5):804-13.

17. Brummett BH, Helms MJ, Dahlstrom WG, Siegler IC. Prediction of all-cause mortality by the Minnesota Multiphasic Personality Inventory Optimism-Pessimism Scale scores: study of a college sample during a 40-year follow-up period. *Mayo Clinic Proceedings* 2006;81(12):1541-4.

18. Kubzansky LD, Sparrow D, Vokonas P, Kawachi I. Is the glass half empty or half full? A prospective study of optimism and coronary heart disease in the normative aging study. *Psychosomatic Medicine* 2001;63(6):910-6.

19. Tindle HA, Chang YF, Kuller LH, Manson JE, Robinson JG, Rosal MC, Siegle GJ, Matthews KA. Optimism, cynical hostility, and incident coronary heart disease and mortality in the Women's Health Initiative. *Circulation* 2009;120(8):656-62.

20. Kubzansky LD, Wright RJ, Cohen S, Weiss S, Rosner B, Sparrow D. Breathing easy: a prospective study of optimism and pulmonary function in the normative aging study. *Annals of Behavioral Medicine* 2002;24(4):345-53.

21. Buchanan GM, Gardenswartz CAR, Seligman MEP. Physical Health Following a Cognitive Behavioral Intervention. *Prevention & Treatment* 1999;2(1):10.

22. Gordon RA. Attributional style and athletic performance: Strategic optimism and defensive pessimism. *Psychology of Sport and Exercise* 2008; 9(3):336-350.

23. Seery MD, Leo RJ, Holman EA, Silver RC. Lifetime exposure to adversity predicts functional impairment and healthcare utilization among individuals with chronic back pain. *Pain* 2010;150(3):507-15.

24. Headey B, Muffels R, Wagner GG. Long-running German panel survey shows that personal and economic choices, not just genes, matter for happiness. *Proceedings of the National Academy of Sciences of the United States of America* 2010;107(42):17922-6.

25. The pursuit of happiness. *New Scientist* 2003;180(2415):40-43.

26. *TD Small Business Happiness Index*, 2010.

27. Lyubomirsky S, Tkach C, Sheldon KM. Pursuing sustained happiness through random acts of kindness and counting one's blessings: Tests of two six-week interventions. In Lyubomirsky S, Sheldon KM, Schkade D. Pursuing happiness: The architecture of sustainable change. *Review of General Psychology* 2005; 9(2):111-131.

28. Emmons RA, McCullough ME. Counting blessings versus burdens: an experimental investigation of gratitude and subjective well-being in daily life. *Journal of Personality and Social Psychology* 2003;84(2):377-89.

29. Floyd K, Mikkelson AC, Tafoya MA, Farinelli L, La Valley AG, Judd J, Haynes MT, Davis KL, Wilson J. Human affection exchange: XIII. Affectionate communication accelerates neuroendocrine stress recovery. *Health Communication* 2007;22(2):123-32.